MW01532928

FITNESS AND FAITH

FITNESS
and
FAITH

The Complete Book of Health
for the Whole Person

DR. PAUL BRYNTESON, D.P.E.

Exercise Physiologist
Director, Health Fitness Program
Oral Roberts University

DONNA BRYNTESON, R.N., B.S.N.

Registered Nurse, Student Health Clinic
Oral Roberts University

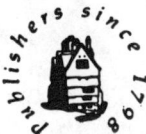

Publishers since 1798

Thomas Nelson Publishers
Nashville • Camden • New York

Copyright © 1985 by Paul Brynteson and Donna Brynteson

All rights reserved. Written permission must be secured from the publisher to use or reproduce any part of this book, except for brief quotations in critical reviews or articles.

Published in Nashville, Tennessee, by Thomas Nelson, Inc. and distributed in Canada by Lawson Falle, Ltd., Cambridge, Ontario.

Printed in the United States of America.

Unless otherwise noted, the Bible version used in this publication is THE NEW KING JAMES VERSION. Copyright © 1979, 1980, 1982, Thomas Nelson, Inc., Publishers.

Scripture quotations noted NASB are from the New American Standard Bible, © The Lockman Foundation 1960, 1962, 1963, 1968, 1971, 1972, 1973, 1975, 1977, and are used by permission.

Scripture quotations noted Amplified are from The Amplified New Testament, copyright © 1954, 1958 by the Lockman Foundation and used by permission.

Scripture quotations noted NIV are from The Holy Bible: New International Version. Copyright © 1978 by the New York International Bible Society. Used by permission of Zondervan Bible Publishers.

Scripture quotations noted TLB are from the The Living Bible (Wheaton, Illinois: Tyndale House Publishers, 1971) and are used by permission.

Scripture quotations noted Phillips are from J. B. Phillips: THE NEW TESTAMENT IN MODERN ENGLISH, revised edition. © J. B. Phillips 1958, 1960, 1972. Used by permission of Macmillan Publishing Co., Inc.

Library of Congress Cataloging in Publication Data

Brynteson, Paul.
  Fitness and faith.

  Bibliography: p. 211
  1. Health. 2. Christian life. 3. Aerobic exercises.
4. Nutrition. 5. Holistic medicine. I. Brynteson,
Donna. II. Title.
RA766.B935   1985   613   85-8902
ISBN 0-8407-5920-7

To our children,
Timothy and Deborah—
two gifts from God.

Contents

Part II: Exercise Your Way to Better Health

Figures

Tables

Preface

The Bible teaches us that "My people are destroyed for lack of knowledge" (Hos. 4:6). If we are to live lives of complete health and well-being, we must have accurate knowledge on which to base decisions of action. More and more people are becoming health conscious and are seeking knowledge about sound health practices. Unfortunately, much misinformation is being published today. As stated by Daniel long ago, "Many shall run to and fro, and knowledge shall increase" (Dan. 12:4). Today, we need sound knowledge to guide us into healthy lifestyles.

The knowledge we use to make quality decisions about our individual lifestyles must come from the information we acquire as we study the Scriptures and from the discoveries of medical science. To be completely healthy, we must follow both spiritual and natural laws. God has created and established both.

This book presents scriptural and scientific knowledge as a basis for developing a healthy lifestyle. Practical guidelines are also provided on how to implement a lifestyle of complete health—physical, spiritual, and emotional. The information in this book is based upon twenty years of university research, teaching, directing health and fitness programs, and personal experience. It has worked for thousands—it has worked for us—it has worked for our entire family. It can work for you.

Introduction

At the conclusion of a seminar I had given on health and fitness, an overweight man in his fifties approached me and began relating his various health problems. He told of his high blood pressure, for which he took medication prescribed by his physician; he often had chest pain, when he would exert himself or was tense; and he had almost constant back pain, for which he was treated regularly by his chiropractor.

He was currently on one of the new diets, one that had worked for a friend. He had tried many diets that were successful for a while, but eventually he would regain all the weight. Further, he had sought prayer for healing at his church; yet, as he shared his problems, I could sense his despair, discouragement, and fear for the future. Nothing seemed to work permanently.

If this case were an isolated one, I could pass it off as one man's problem. However, it is not. Everywhere, people express the same concern and worry about their health. This is especially true of persons over age forty who are beginning to experience nagging problems of poor health. "What should I do?" they ask. "How can I become healthier? I'm looking forward to the freedom of retirement, but rather than freedom I'll be imprisoned by my own poor health."

Regardless of how inviting the picture is painted of heaven with its mansions, lack of sickness, streets of gold, presence of Jesus, and so forth, earth, with all its problems, still attracts us. We don't want to leave it without a struggle. Consequently, whether or not believers in eternal life, people search for health, perhaps for different motives, but still the quest is very real.

Historical Search for Health

People have always searched for health. In 1513, Ponce de Leon, at fifty-three years of age, organized and led an expedition in search of the fountain of youth in the New World. He believed in the legend of a fountain that, when bathed in, would restore youth, vigor, and beauty. Instead of finding it, he discovered Florida and died after he was shot by an Indian's arrow.

Centuries earlier, during the time of Confucius, Chinese emperors hired alchemists to mix doses of gold and mercury into a solution to be drunk because these metals appeared not to tarnish. Unfortunately, mercury is poisonous and caused death rather than longevity. The ancient Egyptians and Romans ate large quantities of garlic to lengthen their lives. Europeans tried a variety of roots and insects.

The ancient Greeks placed great value on health and fitness. Greek teachers emphasized exercise, good nutrition, sanitation, and discipline. The Old Testament Scriptures tied sound health practices to religious laws, especially in sanitation, cleanliness, and diet.

The late nineteenth century, in the United States, saw a great migration to the West. Many people went to discover gold or to start a new life, but historians estimate that at least 25 percent and perhaps as high as 50 percent went to the West, particularly the Southwest, in search of health.

Many people have searched for health in the form of medicines, tonics, and special foods. In the past opium preparations have frequently been taken as painkillers with the result that large numbers of unsuspecting people became addicted. The same was true for "medicinal liquids" taken to soothe the nerves and calm the stomach. Such liquids usually contained large amounts of alcohol and often led to alcoholism in many who innocently used them. It has even been reported that in the late 1800s when a current popular soft drink was first developed, it contained cocaine.

The Current Health Search

Today the search for health seems to have intensified. Of the books on the weekly Top Ten best-selling list, usually two or three are health-related books, usually extolling some new diet. In fact, in 1982 an estimated $50 million was spent in the United States on diet, exercise, and health books. However, that is a small amount compared to the amount spent for all diet, exercise, and health-related expenditures, as indicated by the following figures.

Entrepreneurs have cashed in on the search for health and are promoting various products that promise to improve health. Scarcely a day goes by that we don't read several of the following claims in relation to some product: "The easy way to health," "Lose weight without diet or exercise," "Recommended by a leading medical center." Although exercise has clearly been demonstrated to be beneficial to health, products are be-

PRODUCT	DOLLARS SPENT IN 1980
Diet drinks	6 billion
Exercise clothes	5 billion
Health foods	3 billion
Health clubs	3 billion
Bottled water	2 billion
Vitamins	2 billion
Company fitness programs	2 billion
Sports medicine	2 billion
Swimming	1 billion
Sports shoes	1 billion
Bikes	1 billion
Cosmetic surgery	1 billion
Skiing	570 million
Golf	480 million
Stationary bikes	400 million
Tennis	340 million
Barbells/weights	200 million
Diet pills	200 million
Baseball	160 million
Roller skates	140 million
Dance/exercise programs	40 million

Taken from *Time*, Nov. 2, 1981, p. 103.

ing sold for exercise purposes with the false claims that five minutes per day on a piece of equipment are equivalent to thirty minutes of jogging!

Numerous diet pills, diet aids, body wraps, and electrical stimulation devices are being promoted as beneficial for rapid weight loss—one pound or more per day. If anyone is searching for health, these are sure-fire ways not to obtain it, since any program that recommends more than one to three pounds weight loss per week is suspect and probably doesn't work or is detrimental to health. If it does work, the weight loss is water that will be rapidly regained.

Currently a "fountain of youth" drug is being promoted. Claims have been made that it can remove wrinkles, tighten sagging skin, unclog arteries, increase energy, make you feel thirty years younger, add years to your life, and make you healthier. It sounds good, doesn't it? The interesting fact is that the researchers who pioneered the drug discount such claims and assert that the only persons benefiting from the sale of the drug are those manufacturing and selling it. Be suspicious of any advertisement that claims a quick and easy way to health.

The search for health has led in many directions. Some of the experiments have helped to achieve improved health, some have had no effect other than to waste time and money, and some have actually caused death. Some people have stood on God's Word, confessed their health, and been healed. Other have died with their confessions on their lips. What are the reliable factors that can increase health and longevity? Is there something individuals can do to have optimal health to enjoy life? These are some of the questions I will answer in the following chapters. Sincere people are confused; that confusion can be eliminated.

Part I

Spiritual Dimensions of Health

1

God's Wish for Our Health

One of the fundamental questions a Christian asks is, What is God's will for my life? This question pertains to life in general as well as to specifics. What should my vocation in life be? Whom should I marry? Where should I live? Should I buy a particular car?

But what of the question, Does God want me to be healthy? Just what do the Scriptures tell us concerning His will and our health? In one crucial passage, God, speaking through John, said, "Beloved, I wish above all things that thou mayest prosper and be in health, even as thy soul prospereth" (3 John 2).

That verse has three very important parts. In the first place God said, "Above all things...be in health." There can be no room for misinterpretation. God's will for us is to be healthy. This is not just a passing desire on God's part, but a desire for our good health as a high priority—"above all things."

Second, and very importantly, God doesn't force His will upon us. "Beloved, I wish," indicates the desire of His heart. He *wishes* for us, He *wants* for us, He *desires* that we be in health; but He will not force health upon us. It is our decision to follow a lifestyle that leads to the health He wishes for us. Many of us go through life wishing. We wish for a new car, a new home, a husband or wife, friends, a better job. Unfortunately, wishing alone won't solve the problem. A wish must be followed with action and self-discipline in order for the wish to come true. Wishing for good health is a start—but it must be followed with appropriate behavior.

The third aspect of the verse puts His wish for us in perspective. The phrase, "as your soul prospers," signifies that God's top priority is the salvation of our souls. First and foremost we must accept Christ as Lord and Savior and become new individuals in Christ. But after salvation, God desires for us to be healthy.

What Kind of Health Does God Wish for Us?

Although we may not be able to define exactly what health is, we can usually identify the effects of poor health. Some people experience frequent, recurring illnesses that cause them to be hospitalized. Others suffer from less severe problems that prevent their going about their normal daily activities for a period of time. Most of us experience a feeling of being unwell at some point in our lives.

In the economic arena, the effects of poor health are becoming vividly clear. In 1980, the federal government spent $70.9 billion in health care, up 17 percent from 1979. This expenditure represents the third-largest expenditure in the federal budget, right after defense and social security. General Motors spends more on health benefits for its employees than it does on buying steel for making cars. In 1980, the company spent $1.5 billion financing health care for its employees. This amount, in turn, adds $315.23 to the price of each new car. Poor health is expensive for everyone.

The increasing cost of poor health can also be seen in the total United States' expenditure on health. The total health-care cost has increased from $11 billion in 1950 to $275 billion in 1981 (see Fig. 1.1).

For many years *health* has been considered by most people as "absence of disease." If a person was not sick or had no disease, the individual was said to be healthy. But I believe God intends for us to possess more health than simply absence of disease. Suppose you view two persons, neither of whom is sick. Being free from disease, they are considered healthy. One person is overweight, is often tense and anxious, and has difficulty walking up a flight of stairs without getting out of breath. The other is normal weight, is physically fit, has energy to enjoy numerous activities after a day's work, and is also happy and relaxed. Both have an outward freedom from disease, but they differ significantly in their quality of life and are not really in equally good health.

Just as wealth is more than absence of poverty, happiness is more than absence of sorrow, and being born again is more than absence of sin; health is far more than absence of disease. The health that God desires for us is not just enough health to get by. His desire is that we have optimal living—freedom from diseases *plus* the possession of those important positive health attributes that allow us to live lives of quality and quantity. Jesus spoke of this optimal life when He said, "I have come that they may have life, and that they may have it more abundantly" (John 10:10).

Billions
of
Dollars

275–
250–
225–
200–
175–
150–
125–
100–
75–
50–
25–

1950   1960   1970   1980

Years

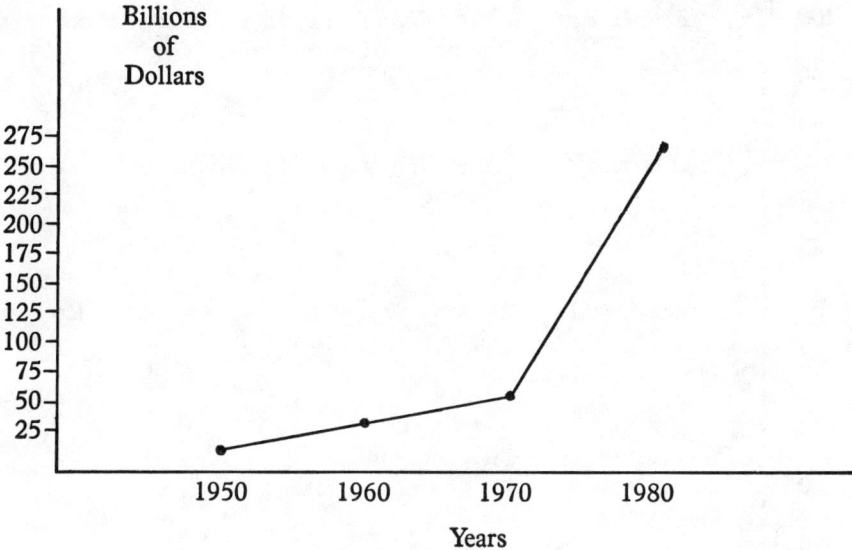

Fig. 1.1. Total Health-care Costs in United States

The Health Continuum

The state of your health can be described in terms of a continuum, a range from very poor health to optimal health. You exist at some point on the continuum and have the capability by choice of moving up or down. An example of such a continuum appears below.

Freedom from disease means that you have health, but that is only 50 percent of what God has intended for you. To have good or optimal health, you must possess additional positive health qualities that result in fitness. Then and only then do you possess sufficient health to stay healthy, resist diseases, enjoy life, and be a glorious temple of the Holy Spirit. God's desire is for you to have optimal health. Where you are on the health continuum depends primarily on you and your lifestyle.

The road to average health is not difficult to follow. Average health is easy to obtain and quite easy to keep. It involves adhering to basic habits such as sanitation, safety, adequate rest and nutrition, having your vaccinations updated, and so on. The road to optimal health, however, is more of an uphill challenge. It requires more of a lifestyle commitment on your part—a bigger seed to plant. It means daily exercise, good nutrition habits, body fat control, meditation on God's Word, and avoidance of alcohol, tobacco, and drugs. With this kind of lifestyle, positive

100	Optimal Health	Possession of an excellent amount of all the positive health qualities
90		
80		
70	Good Health	Possession of several positive health qualities
60		
50	Normal Health	Absence of disease, but possession of few of the positive health qualities
40		
30		
20	Poor Health	Sick quite often
10		
0	Very Poor Health	Bedridden most of the time

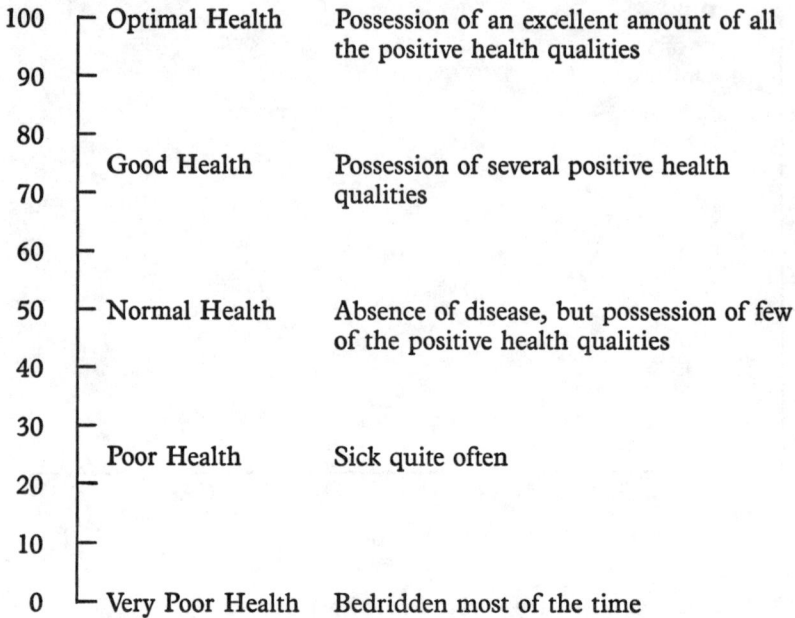

health qualities of good fitness and good body composition will result which, in turn, will help you resist disease and add enjoyment to life. You will be able to live life to its fullest.

Why Optimal Health?

For a number of reasons, God wishes us to have optimal health. First, God loves us (see John 3:16). We are His creation, precious in His sight (see Isa. 43:4). God knows that an abundant life will be difficult for us to achieve without optimal health. So foremost in God's view are His love for us and His desire that we be happy and healthy. God is good and wants good things for His creation.

Second, our bodies are the Lord's property in which the spirit of God lives. "Do you not know...you are not your own? For you are bought at a price" (1 Cor. 6:19–20). When God created Adam from the elements of the earth, he was lifeless until the Lord God "breathed into his nostrils the breath of life; and man became a living being" (Gen. 2:7). Each of us is an earthen vessel in which the spirit of God lives.

However, we are far more than earthen vessels; we are His temples. "Do you not know that you are the temple of God and that the Spirit of God dwells in you?" (1 Cor. 3:16). Many people have a low evaluation of themselves and their bodies, but that is not in keeping with God's view.

He sees each of us as His temple—the home on earth in which He lives and dwells. So why should we have low esteem of our bodies?

What kind of temple does God desire to live in? Fortunately, we don't have to guess or speculate on this point since God gave His blueprint for the temple in the Old Testament. It was built by King Solomon and was one of the wonders of the ancient world. It took seven years to build; it was made with the best materials in the known world, perfectly fitted together, and "the whole temple he overlaid with gold" (1 Kings 6:22).

With the coming of Christ and the new covenant, God proclaimed that now His people are His temple. His people are equated with the old covenant temple as His dwelling place. God wants to take up residency in a temple worthy of His occupancy—a body that is without sin, that is pure, spotless, and healthy. "Therefore glorify God in your body and in your spirit, which are God's" (1 Cor. 6:20). We must follow a lifestyle of health and fitness so that God can be glorified through our bodies.

Third, God wants us healthy so we can serve Him and do His work here on earth. The Great Commission charges us to go into all the world and preach the Good News; we are to be the light on the hill, we are to serve others, and we are to let Christ live through us. We cannot be as effective as possible without optimal health.

Optimal Health and Age

We often associate health with youth. We are programmed to accept youth as being a time of health and the middle and older years as a time when we lose our health, fitness, and vigor. We begin to take it easy, slow down, rest more, and accept more aches and pains.

But God's will for our abundant health is not just when we are young. Our health is to be optimal until we meet the Lord either through the Rapture or through death. First Thessalonians 5:23 states, "May your whole spirit, soul, and body be preserved blameless at the coming of our Lord Jesus Christ." Once again we see the priority—spirit first, then soul and body. Salvation comes first. But note the key word *blameless*. Our bodies are to be blameless until we leave this world. Optimal health is God's will for us for our *entire* lifetimes.

In the fifth chapter of Genesis we are told of people who lived to be 800 to 900 years old. However, in the sixth chapter and thereafter we see a dramatic change. We read, "My Spirit shall not strive with man forever, for he is indeed flesh; yet his days shall be one hundred and twenty years" (Gen. 6:3). God's original plan of a life expectancy of 120 years seems to still apply today. Geneticist Leonard Hayflick has stated that on the basis of his research on cell division and deterioration, man could expect a life span of 110 to 120 years. He reports that human cells in a perfect environment continue to divide until they stop dividing and die according to their genetic code. No disease or sickness caused them to stop.

Could it be that God's will is for optimal health, a blameless spirit, soul, and body, until the time that God will take us home—as He did with Moses? Moses was one hundred and twenty years old when he died. "His eyes were not dim nor his natural vigor abated" (Deut. 34:7). Moses possessed blameless, optimal health until God took him home. The Bible says, "The righteous will flourish like a palm tree...they will still bear fruit in old age, they will stay fresh and green" (Ps. 92:12–14 NIV).

The natural response after this discussion on how we should have optimal, blameless health until age 110 to 120 is, "That's not what I see happening! How could God have given us 120 years when most people don't live past 70 or 80?" The modern evidence is mounting that the way we live our lives is significantly affecting our health and that perhaps we could live to 110 or 120 if our lifestyles were consistent with the way God created us to live.

It all begs the question, What should be the lifestyle for optimal health?

Steps You Could Take

1. Memorize and meditate on the following Scriptures: 3 John 2; 1 Corinthians 6:19–20; 1 Corinthians 3:16; and 1 Thessalonians 5:23.

2. Place yourself on the health fitness continuum.
   a. Do you possess positive health qualities of good fitness and body composition?
   b. Can you jog at least three miles without stopping (or cycle six miles or swim eleven hundred meters)?
   c. Can you do at least thirty situps and twenty pushups?

2

Lifestyle and Health

The Changing Lifestyle

Your lifestyle involves your total behavior, twenty-four hours a day, seven days a week, fifty-two weeks of the year. The number of hours you sleep at night, the food you eat, what you drink, where and how you work, how you relate to others, whether or not you exercise, your church attendance and relationship with God, plus everything else you do, reflect your lifestyle.

The way we live today is not the way our forefathers lived. The American lifestyle has changed significantly over the last eighty years. At the turn of the twentieth century, 70 percent of the American population lived in the country and was physically active in food production. They tilled the soil by walking behind a horse-drawn plow, tended animals, built their own homes, and often fought for survival. The food they ate was not processed or refined.

With advanced technology, occupations became less physically demanding. Walking behind a plow for the farmer gave way to riding on a tractor. Walking to school, church, and the grocery store gave way to riding in the automobile. Wood-burning stoves that required chopped wood for fuel evolved to automatic furnaces. Today, 95 percent of our population lives in cities and is accustomed to work-saving devices, such as power lawn mowers, elevators, golf carts, and weed eaters.

The new discoveries and lifestyle changes have been a mixed blessing for health. On the one hand, our longevity has been improving as the following graph reveals.

Years

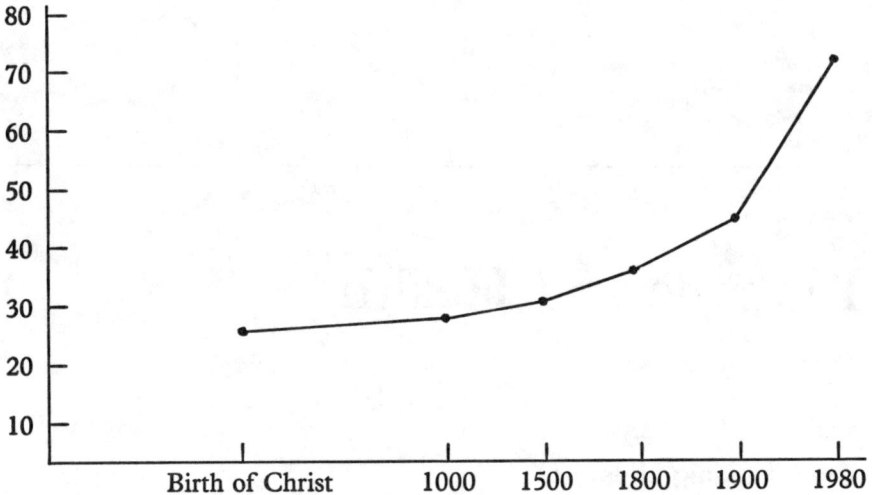

Fig. 2.1. Life Expectancy in the United States from the Birth of
Christ until 1980

In the years from the birth of Christ to 1900, life expectancy at birth
advanced only twenty years (from twenty-five to forty-five). In the eighty
years since 1900, however, life expectancy at birth advanced twenty-
eight years (from forty-five to seventy-three). But before drawing erroneous conclusions attributing the increased life expectancy to lifestyle, we
must look more carefully at the reasons for the increased life span.

During the past one hundred years or so, the medical profession has
made many landmark discoveries. Whereas infectious diseases such as
typhoid fever, smallpox, diphtheria, tuberculosis, scarlet fever, pneumo-
nia, measles, whooping cough, and others caused by microorganisms
killed hundreds of thousands every year in the past, these diseases are almost unheard of today. Medical science has won the battle against infectious diseases through the use of vaccinations and modern medicines. In
1900 the death rate from tuberculosis was 195 per 100,000 persons. Today it is 2 per 100,000 persons. We used to fear outbreaks of polio but
since the Salk vaccine of the 1950s, this disease no longer presents a
threat.

Most of the increase in life expectancy has come from conquering infectious diseases, but not because of major lifestyle changes. Improved
sanitation, vaccinations, antiseptic surgery, and other medical discoveries have all contributed to the increase. In reality, a person at age forty-

five today can expect to live only two or three years longer than a person who made it to age forty-five in 1900.

Major Health Problems Today

The health problems today are different from what they were at the turn of the century. The following table compares the leading causes of death then to those of today.

TABLE 2.1
Leading Causes of Death in the United States
(1900 and 1980)

CAUSE OF DEATH IN 1900	DEATH RATE PER 100,000 POPULATION	CAUSE OF DEATH IN 1980	DEATH RATE PER 100,000 POPULATION
Tuberculosis	195	Heart disease	336
Pneumonia	175	Cancer	181
Diarrhea and enteritis	140	Stroke	85
Heart disease	137	Accidents/nonmotor vehicle	25
Nephritis	89	Pneumonia and influenza	23
Diseases of infancy	72	Motor-vehicle accidents	23
Stroke	72	Diabetes	15
Cancer	64	Cirrhosis of liver	14
Bronchitis	45	Arteriosclerosis	13
Diphtheria	40	Suicide	13
Typhoid fever	31		
Influenza	27		
Polio	26		

Note that the infectious diseases of 1900 have been significantly reduced or are not on the 1980 list at all, thus accounting for the increased life span. On the other hand, the incidence of both heart disease and cancer has virtually tripled since 1900, and those diseases are currently the leading causes of death.

Heart disease, cancer, stroke, diabetes, cirrhosis of the liver, and arteriosclerosis (hardening of the arteries) are considered *degenerative diseases*. They often begin undetected early in life and progressively cause a deterioration in health as we grow older. Often we feel that we are in a state of health because we have no outward symptom of disease. Sometimes the first symptom of a disease like heart disease is also the last, since 40 percent to 50 percent of all heart attack victims die before they reach the hospital after their first heart attack. Coronary arteries can be occluded (obstructed) as much as 50 percent to 70 percent with arteriosclerosis before any symptoms appear. This is why we are emphasizing that health is far more than the outward appearance of freedom from disease. Degenerative diseases are primarily *diseases of lifestyle*.

Lifestyle and Health

It should be evident that the way we live significantly influences our health. The United States Department of Health and Human Services Centers for Disease Control in Atlanta, Georgia, has identified four factors that contribute to the cause of death and disease.

1. *Health system.* The health system is the organization and administration of health care by professionals in our society. It involves doctors, nurses, hospitals, clinics, ambulances, and related health-care personnel and facilities. Occasionally this area is to blame for the death of a person because of misdiagnosis, wrong prescription of medication, or some other neglect or lack of knowledge. The May 1983 issue of *American Druggist* reported that 51 percent of 327 pharmacists surveyed confessed that they had dispensed the wrong medication at least three times during their careers because they couldn't read the physician's handwriting accurately! The problem may also stem from not delivering medical care to locations where it is needed such as rural and low-income areas.

2. *Lifestyle.* As we have previously discussed, the way we live influences our health and can be a major cause of our own death. In some cases we are literally digging our own graves. This idea will be expanded upon later.

3. *Environment.* The evidence is clear that environment (physical, social, economic, and family) can affect our health and may be the primary cause of disease and death. Living and working in high-pollution areas contribute to higher rates of emphysema and lung cancer. Other environmental problems may be stress, toxic materials, transportation, accidents, and so forth.

4. *Genetics.* A person's basic cell structure and characteristics are determined by heredity. The tendency towards heart disease, cancer, hemophilia, sickle cell anemia, diabetes, and certain other diseases may be present at birth. However, heredity alone rarely causes the disease. Usually the tendency interacting with an individual's lifestyle and environment can delay or hasten the prospects of the disease.

The Centers for Disease Control has evaluated the current ten leading causes of death and has allocated the proportion of each of these four contributing factors to the cause of death. The following table reveals their results.

TABLE 2.2
Major Factors Contributing to Death

TEN LEADING CAUSES OF DEATH	PERCENT WHO DIE	FACTOR CONTRIBUTING TO DEATH			
		HEALTH SYSTEM (%)	LIFE-STYLE (%)	ENVIRON-MENT (%)	GENETICS (%)
Heart disease	38.8	12	54	9	28
Cancer	20.9	10	37	24	29
Stroke	9.8	7	50	22	21
All nonvehicle accidents	2.8	14	51	31	4
Influenza and pneumonia	2.7	18	23	20	39
Vehicle accidents	2.7	12	69	18	1
Diabetes	1.8	6	26	0	68
Cirrhosis of liver	1.7	3	70	9	18
Arteriosclerosis	1.6	18	49	8	26
Suicide	1.5	3	60	35	2
Average		10	49	17	24

These statistics clearly place the majority of the responsibility for our health on our own shoulders. Forty-nine percent of the causes of all deaths is due to lifestyle (see Fig. 2.2). Heart disease, stroke, and arteriosclerosis are often combined into a category of cardiovascular disease. These three diseases account for 50.2 percent of all deaths.

In all three cases, lifestyle is the major contributing factor, and when environment is combined with lifestyle, the percentage (over 60 percent) of control we have over cardiovascular diseases is tremendous (see Fig.

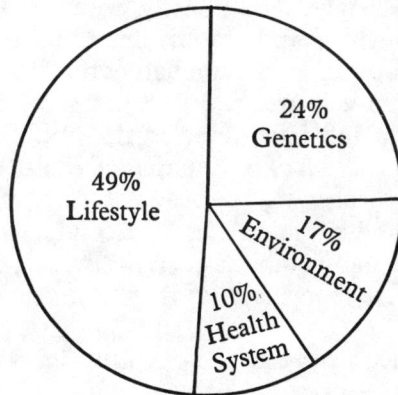

Fig. 2.2. Percentage of the Causes of All Deaths

2.3). In 1979 when Joseph Califano was secretary of the Department of Health, Education, and Welfare, he said, "You, the individual, can do more for your own health and well-being than any doctor, hospital, any drug, any exotic medical device."

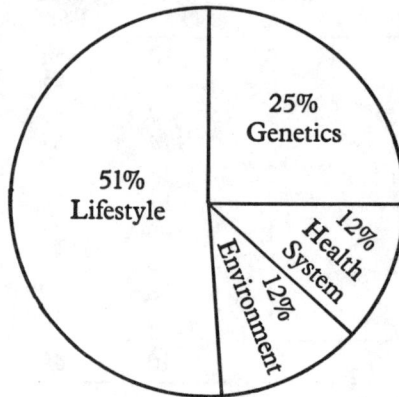

Fig. 2.3. Percentage of the Causes of Cardiovascular Disease

In addition to the statistics from the Centers for Disease Control, other research has shown that lifestyle does significantly affect health. Mormons and Seventh-Day Adventists have been the target of numerous studies because of their healthful lifestyle that emphasizes good diet, exercise, avoidance of alcohol and caffeine, and positive family relationships. Mormons have a cancer rate of only 60 percent of the national average, and Seventh-Day Adventists have a cancer rate of only 50 percent of the national average. Additionally, Seventh-Day Adventists have one-third of the bronchitis and emphysema (both related to smoking), half of the expected heart disease, and half of the diabetes of the national average. They also have a greater life expectancy. Studies comparing death rates in Nevada and Utah revealed that the death rate in Nevada was 35 percent higher for all ages than that of Utah. The primary difference between the two states was the heavy Mormon population in Utah.

Dr. Nedra Belloe and her associates have conducted an ongoing study in California of the relationship between lifestyle characteristics and life expectancy. The seven characteristics they have studied are:

1. Eating three meals per day and avoiding snacks.
2. Eating breakfast every day.
3. Maintaining normal body weight.
4. Exercising moderately.

5. Sleeping seven to eight hours per night.
6. Refraining from smoking.
7. Drinking alcohol in moderation or abstaining completely.

The results have demonstrated that if at age forty-five you follow three or fewer of the above seven lifestyle habits, your life expectancy is another twenty-two years, or age sixty-seven. If, on the other hand, you follow six or seven of the habits, your life expectancy is another thirty-three years, or age seventy-eight. Following these simple lifestyle habits can add eleven years to your life.

Hans Kugler, in his book *Slowing Down the Aging Process*, summarizes some of the key lifestyle behaviors and their health benefits for longevity. Smoking two or more packs of cigarettes per day subtracts eight to nine years from your life, you lose one year for each ten pounds of excess weight you carry, bad nutrition can take six to ten years off your life, and exercise can add six to nine years to your life.

Today are there persons who live long? If there are, what is their lifestyle? Three cultures that appear to have long life expectancies, many over 100 years and some to 120 years and over, are (1) the Vilcabambans of southern Ecuador, (2) the Hunzukuts from the Himalayas of northern Pakistan, and (3) the Caucasian group in Russia between the Black and Caspian seas. All three cultures follow similar lifestyles. Their diets are low in fat, cholesterol, sugar, salt, and calories. They live physically active lives consisting of hard physical work. Finally, all three groups live quiet, peaceful lives with a relaxed environment, few worries, and low stress.

Life insurance companies report that 83 percent of deaths before age sixty-five could have been prevented with a good lifestyle. Studies at the University of Tennessee and at the Massachusetts General Hospital reveal that lifestyle was a major contributing factor in more than 78 percent of the hospital admissions.

What about you and your lifestyle? Is your lifestyle one that is leading to good health? Are you honoring God in your body? What does the Bible have to say about a lifestyle conducive to optimal health?

Steps You Could Take

1. Make sure your immunizations are up-to-date: diphtheria/tetanus—every ten years; polio—lifetime immunity when oral polio series with booster is complete; measles—lifetime immunity if booster given after fifteen months of age; mumps—lifetime immunity with one vaccination; rubella—lifetime immunity with one vaccination; and PPD (TB test)—every three years.

2. After age forty, men should have an annual proctological exam and women an annual pap test. A general physician's evaluation should also be included.

3. Briefly evaluate your lifestyle.
   a. Do you eat three meals a day?
   b. Do you always eat breakfast?
   c. Do you avoid snacks high in sugar and fat?
   d. Are you within ten pounds of a weight desirable for your height?
   e. Do you walk, jog, swim, or cycle without stopping for at least thirty minutes four days per week?
   f. Do you sleep seven to eight hours per night?
   g. Do you smoke or chew tobacco?
   h. Do you use any alcohol or unnecessary drugs?
   i. Do you have any emotional hang-ups?
   The answers to *a* through *f* should be yes; *g*, *h*, and *i* should be no.

4. Is your lifestyle leading you toward optimal health, not only now, but in twenty to forty years from now? To be healthy when you're sixty begin to plant the seeds when you're twenty.

3

Scriptural Guidelines for Health

To assist us in achieving optimal health and abundant life here on earth, God has established two major avenues, spiritual and natural laws, both of which must be followed. Remember, God desires us to be healthy, but He doesn't force health upon us. He provides the means, but we must follow the guidelines. We must develop a lifestyle that results in optimal health.

Sinful Passions Versus the Holy Spirit

Although God has given us spiritual and natural laws to follow to achieve optimal health, we often have inner battles being fought about whether or not we should follow all or any of those laws. The Scriptures teach that it is not in man to direct his own steps (see Jer. 10:23), that we are like sheep who are constantly going astray (see Isa. 53:6), and that the good we know to do we often neglect (see Rom. 7:18–19). Our sinful passions desire one thing, our spirits tell us something else, and the battle goes on in our minds.

Whether the mind decides to follow the Spirit or yield to the desires of the flesh determines not only a person's relationship with God but also his ability to obtain optimal health. "For the mind set on the flesh is death, but the mind set on the spirit is life and peace" (Rom. 8:6 NASB). And we read in Galatians: "Do not be deceived, God is not mocked; for whatever a man sows, this he will also reap. For the one who sows to his own flesh shall from the flesh reap corruption, but the one who sows to the Spirit shall from the Spirit reap eternal life" (6:7–8 NASB). Many of the desires of the flesh lead to poor health. Eating and drinking excessively, smoking, getting angry, being lazy, and indulging in sins are all desires of the flesh that are contrary to the laws of God and very often lead to diseases.

So the first step in being able to follow the spiritual and natural laws God has given for health is to *allow the Holy Spirit to control your mind and heart.* "Walk by the Spirit, and you will not carry out the desire of the flesh" (Gal. 5:16 NASB). This occurs when you commit your life to Jesus Christ and confess Him as Lord and Savior (see Rom. 10:9); you become a new creature with old things leaving your life (see 2 Cor. 5:17). "Now those who belong to Christ Jesus have crucified the flesh with its passions and desires" (Gal. 5:24 NASB).

The second step is to *renew your mind* (see Rom. 12:2). When you become alive in Christ you are born again, but your mind can still overrule the Holy Spirit's guidance. The human mind has been schooled from a human viewpoint. It still has its memories, its emotions, and its own will. Therefore, you must systematically reprogram your mind to think consistently with God's ways. Since God's thoughts are not your thoughts (see Isa. 55:8–9), you must learn His thoughts by daily studying the holy Scriptures. Memorize them, meditate upon them, and then apply them to your life.

> My son, give attention to my words.
> Incline your ear to my sayings.
> Do not let them depart from your sight;
> Keep them in the midst of your heart.
> For they are life to those who find them,
> And health to all their whole body (Prov. 4:20–22 NASB).

Long life, quality of life, and peace are also yours if you keep His commandments (see Prov. 3:1–2).

God's Provisions for Our Health

The first and foremost provision God has made for our health is in the realm of spiritual laws. God is a spirit and so are we. Each of us is given a human spirit, each of us has a soul, and each of us lives in a body. The real core of existence is the spirit. When we yield our spirits to be controlled by His Spirit, we have far fewer problems in this world.

When we become new creatures, we have new power to be used in overcoming the desires of the flesh. Remember, we are not our own; we have been bought with a price. "I beseech you therefore, brethren, by the mercies of God, that you present your bodies a living sacrifice, holy, acceptable to God, which is your reasonable service" (Rom. 12:1). God doesn't take our bodies and their desires; we must take action and present our bodies to Him.

Numerous spiritual laws in the Scriptures assist Christians in their search for health. We will mention only a few of them.

1. *There are health and healing in Christ's sacrifice.* Christ came to earth to live, to die, to resurrect, and to ascend to heaven so we might have total health and healing—spirit, soul, and body. Isaiah 53:5 foretells of this event: "But He was wounded for our transgressions,/He was bruised for our iniquities;/The chastisement for our peace was upon Him,/And by His stripes we are healed." In the New Testament, after these events had taken place, Peter confirmed Isaiah when he said, "Who Himself bore our sins in His own body on the tree, that we, having died to sins, might live for righteousness—by whose stripes you were healed" (1 Pet. 2:24). Accept this provision as yours—that Christ came for your healing and health. Begin to confess it, believe it, and act upon it. Don't accept poor health if you have it. It is not God's desire or will for you.

2. *There are health and healing in Communion.* Communion complements the Atonement since it is by the Communion service that we remember what Christ has done for us through the Atonement. When we partake of the wine, we remember the blood shed by Christ for the salvation of our souls; when we partake of the bread, we are reminded of the body of Christ broken for the healing of our bodies. The body and blood of Christ are life-giving. Our faith is rekindled. Our expectations are heightened, and in persons with that attitude, healing can result. Throughout church history many testimonies have been given by persons whose bodies were healed while taking Communion. In fact, the ancients called Communion "the medicine of immortality."

On the other hand, there is judgment in Communion. We must partake of the bread and wine with the proper attitude and spirit.

> Therefore whoever eats this bread or drinks this cup of the Lord in an unworthy manner will be guilty of the body and blood of the Lord. But let a man examine himself, and so let him eat of that bread and drink of that cup. For he who eats and drinks in an unworthy manner eats and drinks judgment to himself, not discerning the Lord's body. For this reason many are weak and sick among you, and many sleep (1 Cor. 11:27–30).

We should examine our attitudes and spirits when we take Communion, and we should accept His complete salvation and His total health for us as we partake.

3. *There are health and healing in prayer.* Numerous scriptural references concern healing and prayer. We can receive healing for ourselves as we pray for others: "Pray for one another, so that you may be healed" (James 5:16 NASB). Therefore, we shouldn't think only of our own problems when we pray. We must pray for others.

4. *There is healing through the anointing with oil and the laying on of hands.*

> Is any one among you sick? Let him call for the elders of the church, and let them pray over him, anointing him with oil in the name of the Lord. And the prayer of faith will save the sick, and the Lord will raise him up. And if he has committed sins, he will be forgiven (James 5:14–15).

In this connection, the New Testament speaks of the laying on of hands (see Mark 16:18) and the gifts of healings (see 1 Cor. 12:9). The Bible is full of accounts in which Christ, and later His followers, prayed for persons and they were healed. This has continued for the past two thousand years. God never changes (see Mal. 3:6).

If you have a health problem, follow those Scriptures. Pray for others, have others anoint you with oil and pray with you, and have hands laid upon you for healing.

Faith is the foundation of health and healing through spiritual laws. In order to appropriate God's spiritual laws in our lives for health and healing, faith is basic—the foundation, the starting point. "But without faith it is impossible to please Him" (Heb. 11:6). Faith, however, without corresponding action is of little value. James wrote, "Faith by itself, if it does not have works, is dead" (James 2:17). We are saved by faith together with the action of confession: "If you confess with your mouth the Lord Jesus and believe in your heart that God has raised Him from the dead, you will be saved" (Rom. 10:9).

To have the faith necessary to follow God's spiritual laws first requires knowledge of them. To discover the spiritual laws we must study the Scriptures: "So then faith comes by hearing, and hearing by the word of God" (Rom. 10:17). We need to establish the practice of daily Bible reading and meditation.

Biblical Behavior Pattern for Our Health

When God created the world He did so in a precise way. He set in motion exacting laws that give order to the universe. The planets revolve around the sun in a specific pattern. The earth rotates on its axis to give us day and night. Seasons result from the tilting of the earth. Gravity keeps objects and people from floating away from the earth.

We also are precisely made and governed by natural laws. However, there is one difference between people and the rest of the creation. We can choose to follow the natural laws and reap the benefits, or we can reject the natural laws and suffer the consequences. God created us and gave us freedom of choice. Many Christians reject the natural laws God

has established and then seek to put in motion the spiritual laws to coun-
teract the problems caused by not following the natural laws. The Scriptures clearly indicate that this behavior is not part of God's plan for us
and it is not acceptable to God.

How many of us tempt God by claiming health and healing through
scriptural promises but are defying the personal behavior that God also
prescribed? At least seven natural laws must be followed to develop and
maintain optimal halth. Violation of any of the laws leads to health problems sooner or later.

1. *Rest.* The Scriptures tell us that in six days God created the universe and all there is in it and He rested on the seventh (see Gen. 2:2).
God commanded that we should follow His example and rest on the Sabbath (see Exod. 20:9–11). In fact, we are commanded to rest even during
the busiest time of the year (see Exod. 34:21). Jesus also exhorted His
disciples to rest after a time when they had been busy (see Mark 6:31).
Our bodies were created to take a break at least one day per week. Therefore, to have optimal health, we must follow God's commandment and
take a sabbath every week to rest, relax, and renew mind and spirit.

Additionally, we need an adequate amount of daily rest. Research on
sleep indicates we need six to eight hours of good sleep each night to
provide the rest our bodies need. The psalmist tells us, "It is vain for
you to rise up early, /To retire late" (Ps. 127:2 NASB). We need to plan our
daily routine so we get the sleep we need each night.

2. *Avoidance of smoking, alcohol, and other drugs.* Our bodies were not
made to be smokestacks. Until the surgeon general's report in 1962
warning of the danger of smoking, most persons did not consider smoking to be a serious problem. About seventy thousand persons die each
year from lung cancer, and 90 percent of them are smokers. Smoking
also causes the heart to beat faster, promotes irregular pulse, and raises
blood pressure. It is one of the leading factors contributing to heart disease. For every fatal heart attack in a nonsmoking man under age fifty,
men who smoke more than one pack a day account for sixteen.

Alcohol consumption also leads to various problems. More than half
the traffic fatalities involve people who have been drinking. Cirrhosis of
the liver is caused by alcohol consumption and is one of the top ten leading causes of death. When all the problems related to alcohol are combined, it becomes the third leading cause of death, just behind heart
disease and cancer. The Scriptures warn us that the heavy drinker will
come to poverty (see Prov. 23:21) and that the drunkard shall not inherit
the kingdom of God (see 1 Cor. 6:10).

3. *Safety.* Good safety habits are often overlooked as a natural law. Unfortunately, accidents are the leading cause of death in persons under age

thirty-nine, and accidents claim more lives from ages fifteen to twenty-four than all other deaths combined. Accidents not only claim lives but also result in many crippling injuries. Many young people have been paralyzed from the waist down (paraplegic) or from the neck down (quadriplegic) because they hit a rock while diving in a lake and broke their necks. God wants us to use good common sense and to be safety conscious to prevent accidents. We should be sensitive to the leading of the Holy Spirit in our lives. We should heed the warnings He gives as He may be warning that there is danger ahead if we do what we're considering.

4. *Exercise.* Exercise has clearly come to the forefront as an important natural law that must be followed to achieve optimal health. A scriptural reference that has been misinterpreted by many Christians and used as an excuse not to exercise is 1 Timothy 4:8. In the Amplified Bible the verse states, "For physical training is of some value." First of all, note "some value." It doesn't say no value.

Second, considering the lifestyle in A.D. 50 that consisted of walking, hard physical work, and no labor-saving devices, Paul could say to Timothy that physical training is of some value but not a lot of value. They probably got all the exercise they needed in their daily routines. I believe he would have worded it differently if he had written it during our sedentary era.

Third, we must look at the context of the verse. Paul is comparing physical exercise with spiritual exercise. In comparison, physical exercise is of less importance, since its value is only for this life. Spiritual exercise is of greater value because it benefits us not only in this life but also in the life to come. I couldn't agree more. Since exercise is so important for optimal health, I will discuss it extensively in chapters 5 through 12.

5. *Body fat control.* Our bodies were made to have some fat on them but not too much. Far too many people in America have too much body fat. An obese person has twelve times the death rate from heart disease, stroke, and diabetes than the person of normal weight. The Scriptures also tell us that excess fat is undesirable: "Do not be with heavy drinkers of wine, /Or with gluttonous eaters of meat; /For the heavy drinker and the glutton will come to poverty" (Prov. 23:20–21 NASB). Christians have often been quick to condemn the drunkard and ignore the glutton. The Scriptures seem not to distinguish between them. I will discuss the problem of excess body fat and how to control it in chapters 13 through 15.

6. *Diet.* Our bodies were formed from the dust of the earth, and they contain specific quantities of elements that need constant replacement.

Through the food we eat we restore the elements and nutrients needed for the cells to function properly. According to Scriptures, we are to put a knife to our throats if we have great appetites (see Prov. 23:2 NASB), and we are to eat no fat (see Lev. 3:17).

Today research is demonstrating the need to have a good balanced diet and to return to the biblical recommendations. Diet will be discussed in chapters 16 and 17.

7. *Emotional stability.* We cannot disassociate physical health from emotional and spiritual health. Because of the interrelatedness of the mind, body, and spirit, no one can achieve optimal health physically until the mind and the spirit are also healthy. Medical science has demonstrated that anxiety, depression, worry, and fear can lead to physical disorders. Some authorities estimate that 30 percent to 50 percent of physicians' patients have *psychosomatic* ailments (physical disorders due to mental or spiritual worries). An optimistic outlook is the first step in developing optimal health. We will discuss this more thoroughly in chapters 18 and 19.

Your Responsibility

Have you been searching for optimal health but it somehow seems to elude you? *You can have optimal health!* You can be free from disease and possess the health qualities essential to keep you free from disease. Although God has made numerous provisions for your health, you have a responsibility to apply those provisions to your life. God won't do it for you.

Steps You Could Take

1. Make Jesus Christ Lord and Savior of your life.

2. Begin to renew your mind by meditating at least thirty minutes every day on God's Word.

3. Accept God's provisions for your health and healing.

4. Study the rest of this book thoroughly so you can effectively follow God's natural laws of exercise, weight control, nutrition, and stress management.

4

Our Responsibility for Health

To the graduating class of 1976 from Oral Roberts University, the founder and president gave this charge:

You do what you can do,
Let God do what He can do,
But don't you try to do what only God can do,
And don't you expect God to do what you're supposed to do.

God has given us responsibility for our health. He wishes above all things for us to be healthy, and He has made provisions for our health through natural and spiritual laws. But we must apply those laws to our lives. Why do some people say, "I really should quit smoking," or "I know I need to lose weight," or "I should get more exercise," yet continue the same hazardous lifestyle and ignore the natural laws as if nothing will happen to them? How does God view the smoker who prays to God to heal his lung cancer? God in His grace can heal the lungs, but people "tempt" God with such prayers (see Matt. 4:7). He is probably not very receptive to them. We must do our part first, then expect God to do His part.

Numerous accounts in the Scriptures demonstrate God doing His part, and man doing his part. God delivered Noah and his family from the Flood, but Noah had to obey God and build the ark. He was saved by natural means. Abraham was given the Promised Land, but he had to make the journey to possess it. The walls of Jericho fell down, but the children of Israel had to walk around the city once a day for six days and seven times on the seventh day. Perhaps some of us are ineffective today because we're not fit enough to build the ark, make the journey, or march around the city for seven days.

The Scriptures point out our responsibility for our own health, happiness, and prosperity. The psalmist tells us that whatever we do shall prosper (see Ps. 1:3). Christ spoke the words, "Your faith has made you whole," on several occasions (see Matt. 9:22; Mark 5:34).

In Acts 12 is the account of Peter's escape from prison. His Christian friends fervently prayed for his release from the moment he was apprehended. When the angel of the Lord appeared to release Peter, the angel caused the chains to fall off, opened the locked gates, and kept the guards asleep. All these things Peter could not do. But what Peter could do, he did. He obeyed when he was told, "Gird yourself, put on your shoes and your coat, and follow me." God could have supernaturally transported Peter from the jail to the home where the people were praying for him, but He didn't. God did His part and Peter had to do his.

A "Want To" Attitude

The most important responsibility in any program of health and fitness involves attitude. Little benefit is going to be achieved unless a person has an intrinsic desire—a deep "want to" within—to develop and maintain personal health and fitness. The desire must be present to have more than the absence-of-disease kind of health. The desire must be to have optimal health and discipline to make necessary lifestyle changes.

Many people claim that they want to improve their health and fitness, but it is often for extrinsic reasons. For example, a college or university student in a physical education class may want to lose weight in order to receive a good grade or pass the class. If that is the only reason the person wants to lose weight, the effectiveness of that program is going to be short-lived. Sometimes a person wants to lose weight to please other people, such as parents, spouse, or children. If that is the incentive to lose weight, the program will die. Other people announce intentions to lose weight and describe how they want to improve health and fitness but make little or no continuous effort to do so. The desire is not sincere; it is only superficial.

Some people want to lose weight and improve their fitness in order to look better. They are not really concerned about health and fitness, but they want to present a good appearance. If that inward motive is strong enough, often a positive result of a program that leads to a good appearance will be good health. That type of motive is an acceptable motivator to diet and exercise. On the other hand, if this desire is so strong that the people do unhealthful things, they may end up looking better but at the cost of damaging their health along the way. This is especially true of those who follow fad diets or excessive fasts.

By far the best motivator to exercise and to control our diets is the acknowledgment that our responsibility is to take care of our bodies. In many young persons this motivation is not strong because they often enjoy good health but not optimal health. Often this motivator does not surface until age forty, fifty, or sixty which, unfortunately, is too late in some cases.

Many people have abused their bodies for ten or twenty years or more. They begin to suffer the result of this abuse, and then they become concerned about health and want to do something about it. Sometimes this resolve comes on the heels of the first heart attack, and it may be too late. Or maybe it is after years of back problems with resultant hospitalization. These people may have difficulty overcoming the years of abuse and neglect of their bodies.

The most effective desire is to really believe the health value of exercise. If we know what it will do for us in our lives, we can be motivated from within because of the yearning for optimal health. It is far easier to develop a good level of health and fitness when we are young than attempting to overcome the years of abusing our bodies and develop fitness when we are older. "I have set before you life and death...choose life in order that you may live" (Deut. 30:19 NASB).

Accurate Knowledge

After people develop a genuine desire to take responsibility for their own health and fitness program, they need accurate knowledge about how to implement such a program. Hosea 4:6 states, "My people are destroyed for lack of knowledge." Nowhere is this truer than in health and fitness. People are always looking for the easy way out; as the old saying goes, "The spirit is willing but the flesh is weak." As a result, they are open and gullible to gimmicks and the easy way to fitness—the pill to quickly shed that unwanted fat or any device or plan that will improve fitness without effort.

A major problem is that everyone claims to be an expert in health, nutrition, and exercise. Over the last few years, most of the books and articles on the topic have not been written by professionally trained persons but rather by individuals jumping on the "health kick" bandwagon. Much false and erroneous information is being published.

Any promoter of health and fitness should meet two prerequisites before presuming to qualify as an expert. First and foremost is academic training. If the person has an academic degree in the area he or she is writing about, the information is more likely to be accurate. A person recommending exercise programs should have an academic degree in exercise physiology. People with this degree have studied the anatomy and physiology of the body and know how best to exercise to develop the body. Just because someone directs a health club, has attended a few fitness clinics, has a well-developed body, or is a physician doesn't mean that person is knowledgeable in exercise physiology.

A person offering advice on diet and nutrition must have had at least some training in biochemistry before presuming to counsel on this highly controversial area. Many of the current best-selling books on diet are written by those with no training in nutrition, and their statements reveal their lack of accurate information. Many of their recommendations are harmful. Numerous people gain much of their nutrition information from such sources and from magazine articles that offer faulty "helpful" hints.

Marsha Hudnall, a registered dietitian and a research associate with the American Council on Science and Health, reviewed the accuracy of nutrition information in nineteen journals that publish nutrition articles. Her findings, published in a story, "Nutrition: Whom Can You Trust?", in the *Tulsa World* on March 7, 1982, revealed that many of the articles presented inaccurate information.

The second prerequisite in evaluating the credentials of the writer or speaker is, Does his life demonstrate that what he says works for him? Heed not the advice of an unfit person, whether that person is a nutritionist, nurse, exercise leader, or physician. Seek out academically trained people who practice personally what they have learned and follow their advice.

Changing Your Lifestyle

Once you have determined you want to have the optimal and abundant health that God wishes, you are ready to begin. Make a commitment to follow a good health program starting today and continue it the *rest of your life*. This is not a crash program since such programs usually do crash. This book describes a program that is a lifestyle. Optimal health results from following such a lifestyle for the rest of your life. The following can help you to change your lifestyle permanently.

1. *Be patient.* Don't expect to change all your bad habits overnight and to immediately develop a consistent healthful lifestyle. You will probably backslide occasionally. The faster you attempt to make changes, the more likely you are to run into snags. This is especially true in exercising and in changing your eating habits.

Those who haven't jogged in years may become motivated to exercise, and they begin jogging too soon and injure a joint, which puts a damper on exercise for perhaps weeks or months. Begin gradually. If you haven't exercised in twenty years, don't expect fitness to be developed in twenty days. It may take twenty months! But it will be developed if you don't give up. "Let us not grow weary while doing good, for in due season we shall reap if we do not lose heart" (Gal. 6:9).

2. *Change one thing at a time.* Perhaps you have identified several life-style changes you need to make. Begin a one-month program to change one thing at a time. The first month, if you aren't already doing it, meditate thirty minutes on the Scriptures, especially emphasizing the positive Scriptures (see chap. 18). For the second month begin a regularly scheduled exercise program that we will outline in later chapters. The third month, begin to make diet changes. By changing one thing at a time, you will more gradually change your lifestyle, and the change will be more permanent than if you try to change everything at once.

3. *Having fun is not the issue.* We don't follow sound health practices necessarily because they are fun. Many people don't jog because they think it's not any fun or it's boring. That is not the issue. We don't brush our teeth each day, wash our hands before we eat, put money in a savings account, or study before we take a test because these things are fun. We do many things in life because we know and value their long-term benefits. So it is with a healthy lifestyle. Discipline your life to do what is right, not necessarily what feels good. However, we guarantee that in the long run your life will be one of quality and quantity because of a healthy lifestyle.

4. *Don't be embarrassed to exercise.* Many persons are too timid to start an exercise program, jog, or walk in front of others because of what people will say, or they don't want people to see them. If Christ could suffer a shameful death on a cross for your total well-being, the least you can do is care for your body without suffering embarrassment. If you're embarrassed to exercise in front of people, perhaps the timidity is really hidden pride.

5. *Combine the natural and the spiritual.* Healing and optimal health are best achieved when you combine the natural and spiritual laws. When by faith you accept what Christ has done for you, and live a lifestyle consistent with His spiritual and natural laws, you can expect optimal health. "And they overcame him by the blood of the Lamb [God's part] and by the word of their testimony [your part]" (Rev. 12:11).

When the children of Israel fearfully looked at the Red Sea and called on God, God told Moses, "Quit praying and get the people moving! Forward, march!" (Exod. 14:15 TLB).

Steps You Could Take

1. Determine in your heart that you will develop a healthy lifestyle that leads to optimal health and fitness.

2. Determine that you will faithfully and consistently do your part to achieve optimal health and expect God will do His part.

3. Desire to achieve optimal health since you are the temple of God.

4. Select which lifestyle changes you will make in the first month, second month, and so on.

5. Be patient.

Part II

Exercise Your Way to Better Health

5

The Cardiorespiratory System

Function of Cardiorespiratory System

The basic unit of life in the human organism as well as in all other life forms is the cell. More than one trillion cells are in the human body. It would take about forty thousand blood cells to fill the typewriter letter *O*. Every minute about three billion cells in our bodies die and three billion new cells are formed to replace them. What a fantastic body God created for us! "I will praise You for I am fearfully and wonderfully made" (Ps. 139:14).

Every cell has a specific function. Some cells are specialized to cause movement (muscle cells), some are specialized to carry messages (nerve cells), and others are specialized to carry on other functions such as digestion and reproduction. However, for all cells to function, regardless of their structure and purpose, there are four requirements: (1) every cell needs oxygen; (2) every cell needs nutrients (carbohydrates, proteins, fats, vitamins, and minerals); (3) every cell needs water; and (4) every cell needs to get rid of waste products. Of the four requirements, the need for oxygen is the most critical since the body can survive for weeks without food and days without water but only minutes without oxygen.

In order for the cells to receive a constant supply of oxygen, several systems in the body must function together. The cardiorespiratory system is composed of several structural components: (1) heart; (2) lungs and the air-pathways to and from the lungs; and (3) the blood and blood vessels.

The Heart—the Pump of Life

The heart is a muscle with four chambers: two upper chambers (atria) and two lower chambers (ventricles). The heart functions as a pump that provides the force to transport blood to and from the cells. Each time the heart muscle contracts, it creates a pressure that forces blood pulsating in a given direction so oxygen and nutrients can be carried to the cells and back again to the heart to be recirculated. The heart has a tremendous capacity to vary in the number of times it contracts, or beats, per minute. An adult's heart rate may vary from 50 or 80 beats per minute at rest to as high as 180 or 200 beats per minute during maximal exercise.

Table 5.1*
Adult Resting Heart Rate Per Minute

HEALTH FITNESS STANDARD	MEN	WOMEN
Very poor	80 plus	82 plus
Poor	72–80	75–82
Fair	64–72	66–75
Good	50–64	55–66
Excellent	50 or fewer	55 or fewer

*For a person without heart disease

The resting heart rate varies considerably between fit and unfit persons. The preceding table shows that a highly fit person's heart will beat almost half as much as an unfit person's heart. It is much stronger and healthier, and it will respond better when called upon in emergencies. The heart of a person whose resting heart rate is 80 beats per minute will beat 115,200 times per day. The heart of a person whose resting heart rate is 50 beats per minute will beat only 72,000 times per day. His heart beats 43,200 fewer times per day than that of the unfit person. His heart is going to last much longer than the unfit person's. Also, the slower the heart beats, the better the heart muscle itself can receive blood to feed its cells. The heart muscle feeds itself only when it is at rest and not contracting.

The stronger the heart muscle, the more blood that can be pumped and delivered to the cells of the body. A highly fit person's heart can pump twenty-five to thirty quarts of blood per minute at maximum output, whereas an unfit person's heart may pump eight to ten quarts of blood per minute at maximum output. Therefore, all the cells of the highly fit person's body will function more efficiently. They will receive a greater supply of nutrients and will better slough off the waste products. The cells will be better able to handle stresses and combat disease.

Blood Pressure

As the heart contracts, blood is pumped through large arteries of the body to the cells. The ejected blood has a tremendous force behind it, which creates pressure against the artery walls. As the heart relaxes, the pressure against the artery walls decreases.

By means of a sphygmomanometer and a stethoscope, it is possible to determine the blood pressure in the arteries. A cuff is wrapped snugly around the arm just above the elbow. It is inflated until its pressure exceeds the pressure of the blood against the artery wall, which stops the blood flow through the artery. Below the cuff the stethoscope is placed over the brachial artery, then pressure is slowly reduced in the cuff until detection of the first sound of blood passing through the artery. This is the *systolic pressure* and indicates that the pressure exerted by the blood in the artery during contraction of the heart is greater than pressure in the cuff.

The cuff will still partially close the artery when the heart relaxes between contractions. As pressure in the cuff is gradually lowered, a sudden muffling sound is heard through the stethoscope, which indicates that the cuff is no longer shutting off the artery during the resting place of the heartbeat cycle. The pressure at this point is called the *diastolic pressure*.

Normal values for blood pressure range widely. Blood pressure usually increases with age, and this increase is accepted as a normal part of aging. This is not, however, desirable because it may indicate that the vascular system is providing greater resistance to the blood flow due to inelasticity of the arteries.

High blood pressure is called *hypertension*. "Average" blood pressure is considered 120/80, but 100/60 and 140/90 are also normal. Blood pressure varies from hour to hour and person to person. Often the anxiety of a medical examination in a doctor's office elevates blood pressure. In evaluating the pressure a physician must consider all factors before making a diagnosis. High blood pressure has been called the *silent killer* since it often goes undetected and significantly contributes to stroke, heart attack, and kidney failure. Therefore, it is extremely important that you have your blood pressure taken regularly. If it is high, it can be controlled through diet, salt restriction, exercise, relaxation techniques, and perhaps medication.

If we consider only blood pressure, a thirty-five-year-old person with a normal blood pressure of 120/80 can expect to live to age seventy-six. On the other hand, a person with blood pressure 150/100 or greater can expect to live to only sixty. This represents sixteen years of reduced life expectancy. God surely doesn't expect us to lose sixteen years of our life and service to Him because of high blood pressure, especially when something can be done about it. Find out your blood pressure, and then take the corrective lifestyle changes to lower it.

Table 5.2
Resting Systolic Blood Pressure

HEALTH FITNESS STANDARD	UNDER AGE 30	30–60	OVER 60
Very poor	150 plus	160 plus	170 plus
Poor	135–150	140–160	150–170
Fair	125–135	130–140	135–150
Good	115–125	120–130	125–135
Excellent	105–115	105–120	105–125

Coronary Blood Flow

Although tremendous quantities of blood flow through the heart chambers every minute, the heart itself does not receive any nutrients or oxygen from the blood flowing through its chambers. Rather, the heart has its own artery, capillary, and vein system.

The *coronary arteries* are three arteries that supply the blood to the heart muscle. They branch off from the large artery (aorta), leaving the heart within several inches of its beginning. The blood flow through the coronary arteries that supplies the heart muscle itself with oxygen and nutrients is critical. As the skeletal muscles demand more blood with physical activity, the heart muscle also requires a proportional increase in blood.

Table 5.3
Resting Diastolic Blood Pressure

HEALTH FITNESS STANDARD	UNDER AGE 30	30–60	OVER 60
Very poor	97 plus	100 plus	102 plus
Poor	88–97	90–100	92–102
Fair	80–88	82–90	84–92
Good	72–80	74–82	76–84
Excellent	60–72	60–74	60–76

Although the heart is 1/200 of total body weight, it requires 1/20 of the blood pumped from it. When fat (or more accurately, *plaque*) deposits occur in the coronary arteries (*atherosclerosis*), this reduces the flow of blood to the heart muscle. This may present no problem at rest, but as greater and greater demands occur, the supply becomes less and less sufficient.

When the demand of the heart muscle for oxygen is not being met by the coronary blood flow, the area of the heart deficient in oxygen becomes *ischemic* (lack of oxygen). This lack of oxygen can result in *angina pectoris*, a pain in the chest that usually radiates to the left shoulder and arm. However, the pain could also go to the neck and right shoulder or be a discomfort in the upper chest. It is a warning signal and should be heeded. Persons who experience this pain should ease up on whatever they are doing and consult a doctor immediately. Ischemia to the heart muscle can lead to death of the affected heart muscle (*myocardial infarction*), which is more commonly known as a heart attack. The severity of the heart attack depends upon the location and size of the infarction. It may be unnoticed, or it may result in death.

The Electrocardiogram

In the right upper chamber of the heart is a specialized group of heart muscle cells known as the *pacemaker*. This pacemaker initiates the heartbeat by sending out impulses that radiate across the heart and cause it to beat in a regular rhythmical pattern. Normally at rest, the pacemaker sends out fifty to eighty impulses per minute.

The function of the heart can be evaluated by looking at its electrical activity as measured through an *electrocardiogram* (ECG or EKG). Because the heart is a muscle, electrical activity is present when it contracts, and this electrical activity spreads to the surface of the body. The normal flow of electrical impulses through the heart has been recorded and standards have been given. Any deviation of the waves of an electrocardiogram may indicate some specific heart problem. Also, any change in the rhythm of the heartbeat (an *arrhythmia*) may indicate a structural or functional heart defect.

The resting ECG can determine if heart damage exists, but it is not as valuable in detecting underlying heart disease as is the *graded exercise test* (GXT) with ECG. In this test a person walks on a treadmill or pedals a stationary bike until exhausted, and an ECG is monitored during the exercise. It is recommended that all persons over age thirty-five to forty have an exercise ECG test every one to three years and especially before beginning an exercise program.

Breathing

It would be convenient if the oxygen in the air could pass directly through the skin and go to the cells, but our bodies were not created that way. We must inhale in order to bring air into our lungs where the oxygen can diffuse into the blood stream to be transported to the cells, and carbon dioxide can diffuse from the blood into the lungs and leave our bodies when we exhale.

We do not think every time we take a breath; rather, it occurs involuntarily. Our higher brain centers can override the involuntary response in that we can breathe faster, breathe slower, or hold our breath if we choose to do so. However, if we held our breath until we fainted we would involuntarily start breathing again. As the inspired air passes through the passageways to the lungs, it is moistened, cooled or warmed, and cleansed of foreign particles so that the air has a consistent make-up when it arrives in the lungs.

The *diaphragm* is the chief muscle involved in breathing, and it works hard when you exercise. If you exercise more vigorously than you are accustomed to, the constant contraction and relaxation of the diaphragm may lead to a *side ache*. This pain is caused by a lack of oxygen getting to the diaphragm muscle; waste products have built up. You should slow down your exercise intensity since your diaphragm cannot accommodate the excessive demand.

You should not exercise strenuously after a big meal, since when the diaphragm contracts and lowers in the abdominal cavity, it will run into a full stomach. This will limit the breathing capacity, and once again a side ache may result. Also, blood is pooled in the stomach after a meal to aid in the digestion process; therefore, blood is not as readily available for the muscles for heavy exercise. Wait two hours after a heavy meal before exercising. An easy walk after a heavy meal is acceptable.

Asthma is a condition that inhibits large quantities of air from getting into the lungs. In asthma sufferers, the small tubes in the lungs through which the air passes can be constricted, thereby preventing a large flow of air through the tubes to the part of the lungs where the diffusion takes place. In this case, the lung can inhibit the availability of large amounts of oxygen capable of being diffused into the blood stream.

Altitude is another factor that can prohibit large quantities of oxygen from going to the blood stream. At high elevations, the barometric pressure is lower, creating a lower pressure of oxygen. Therefore, the higher the altitude, the less oxygen available to diffuse into the blood stream. It will take six to ten seconds longer to run a mile at 5,200 feet than at sea level.

Blood and Blood Vessels

The blood vessels of the body and the blood are the transportation system that carries oxygen from the lungs to the cells and carbon dioxide from the cells back to the lungs. The oxygen is carried in the blood by the red blood cells and is specifically carried by the iron portion of the *hemoglobin* of the red blood cell. Therefore, it is critically important to have a good source of iron in your diet. The normal hemoglobin for an adult male is about fifteen grams per one hundred milliliters of blood at sea-level conditions and fourteen grams per one hundred milliliters for females. You should have your hemoglobin measured by a physician. Sometimes low hemoglobin can cause you to feel tired and lethargic.

Recently a friend of ours was constantly tired, and she would sleep ten hours at night, but she still had no energy. When her hemoglobin was checked, it was found to be 9.3 grams/100 milliliters rather than the normal 14. She therefore had a 33 percent reduction in oxygen-carrying capacity of her blood. No wonder she felt tired! She was placed on a special diet rich in iron, and within weeks she felt herself again.

The blood vessels that transport oxygen, carbon dioxide, nutrients, and blood components are made up of *arteries* (which carry blood away from the heart), *veins* (which carry blood back to the heart), and *capillaries* (small vessels that connect arteries and veins). Healthy arteries are elastic. When blood is pumped from the heart and flows into the large arteries under very high pressure, the arteries will stretch to accept the blood and help push it to the peripheral vessels. When fatty deposits accumulate inside the larger arteries, the elasticity decreases, and the capacity of these arteries to respond properly to large volumes of blood is diminished. This increased resistance prevents the heart from efficiently pumping blood from its chamber.

The healthy vein is nonelastic. Since the pressure is less in veins and in many cases blood is circulating against gravity back to the heart, the veins have one-way valves to prevent a backflow of blood. Because the valves in the veins are one-way, when muscles contract they aid in squeezing the blood back to the heart. If the vessels become too elastic, the valves do not close tightly, which permits a backflow of blood.

Persons who stand motionless or are on their feet for long periods of time, such as dentists, nurses, and waitresses, are more susceptible to pooling of blood in the veins, and the valves may cease functioning properly and eventually lead to *varicose veins* (enlarged, discolored veins usually in the lower legs). Persons with these jobs should (1) often contract their leg muscles while standing, (2) take breaks and sit down and elevate their legs, and (3) wear support stockings.

Steps You Could Take

1. Measure your resting heart rate. To get a valid resting measure, record your heart rate five days in a row in the morning before you get

out of bed. (Count your heart rate for ten seconds and multiply this value time six.) Record the lowest value. _____ What health fitness category is it? _____

2. What is your systolic blood pressure? _____
   What health fitness category is it? _____
   What is your diastolic blood pressure? _____
   What health fitness category is it? _____

3. If you are over age thirty-five, have a graded exercise test with an ECG. If you are under age thirty-five, but have a history of heart problems or high blood pressure, or have angina pain, also have a graded exercise test with ECG.

4. If you feel tired or lethargic more often than you feel you should, have your hemoglobin evaluated.

6

Risk Factors Related to Cardiovascular Disease

Adaptation

Our bodies have an amazing ability to adapt to factors that influence them, for both the good and the bad. When we travel to higher elevations (greater than 7,500 feet above sea level), over a several-week period our bodies will adapt to the low pressure of oxygen in the air by producing more hemoglobin, thereby increasing oxygen delivery to our cells.

If a person often takes antacids, over a period of time the stomach will adapt by producing more acid. The net effect of the overmedication is a vicious cycle: more stomach acid, more antacids; more antacids, more stomach acid. The same can be said for most medicines.

Since the days of Hippocrates, the father of medicine who lived before the birth of Christ, it has been widely known that that which is used develops and that which is not used wastes away. This principle has been ignored by most people today. If we exercise the heart muscle, it becomes strong and can withstand much wear and tear. If we do not regularly exercise the heart muscle, it becomes weak and inefficient and begins the process of deterioration that may eventually kill us. Even though an individual feels healthy, alert, and fit at age twenty or thirty, the degeneration of the heart muscle may be occurring. Atherosclerosis of the blood vessels begins with the coronary arteries becoming smaller and smaller. After ten or twenty years, symptoms may occur such as shortness of breath after walking up stairs, general fatigue, and mild chest pain after physical activity.

At this point it is not too late to attempt to reverse the deterioration, but all too often we pray for healing and by faith claim that we're not going to have a heart attack. Fine! We must put action with faith, follow God's natural laws, and then begin to change our lifestyles.

Unfortunately, too many persons are losing their lives in their prime because of heart attack. They failed to heed God's natural laws of exercise, diet, stress control, and weight control.

The same principle also applies to the back, by the way. Eighty percent of all Americans suffer from chronic backache; the primary cause is neglect of the back, mainly through lack of exercise but also through poor posture, incorrect sleeping position, and bad sitting habits. These problems will be discussed in chapters 10 and 11.

Also senility, which often occurs with old age, has been attributed to the aging process. In large part, however, it is not old age itself that is the problem but lack of use. If you stop challenging your brain, requiring it to think and solve problems, it falls prey to deterioration from lack of use. Your body organs, including muscles and brain, were not meant to slow down at some magic retirement age of sixty-five. They must continue to be used and exercised to develop and maintain optimal health.

The Making of a Heart Attack

Since heart disease and related cardiovascular problems are the major degenerative diseases that kill Americans, we should specifically examine some of the factors related to them. If we explore ways we can reduce our chances of heart disease, we can live out our life spans with optimal health and serve God effectively throughout our lives.

The underlying cause in 95 percent of cardiovascular disease (heart attack and stroke) is atherosclerosis. Several things happen in the process:

- Artery wall thickens.
- Artery wall loses its elasticity and hardens.
- Several *lipids* (blood fats) deposit on the inner layer of the artery wall. These include cholesterol, triglycerides, phospholipids, and fatty acids.
- Minerals, especially calcium, also deposit on the inner layer of the artery wall.
- The deposits are known as *plaque.*
- The opening in the artery through which the blood passes becomes narrower so that less blood can flow through the artery.
- Circulation is reduced.

The atherosclerotic process takes place largely without symptoms until the arteries are 75 percent occluded (closed). At this point, if the occluded artery is in the heart, chest pain (angina pectoris) may be experienced during physical activity or periods of stress. If the occluded artery is in the brain, brief blackouts, dizzy spells, or tingling in the brain may be experienced. (Incidentally, an EKG stress test can detect when there is about a 50 percent or more occlusion of a coronary artery.)

At one time authorities considered atherosclerosis to be a part of aging and an old person's disease. Medical evidence discovered over the past ten to fifteen years reveals that atherosclerosis is *not* just an old person's disease but begins in young persons and progresses. Autopsies done on Americans killed in the Korean War revealed that 77 percent had some degree of coronary atherosclerosis. This finding was also observed in autopsies of Americans killed in Vietnam. The startling fact was that the average age of these soldiers was twenty-two!

As the arteries continue to narrow because of atherosclerosis, a time will come when blood cannot flow through the artery. The result is a heart attack. If the sealed-off artery supplied a very small part of the heart, especially in the atria, the heart attack may go unnoticed. That results in a "silent heart attack." If the artery supplied a larger portion of the heart, the person may experience any or all of the following symptoms:

- Uncomfortable pressure and fullness in the chest lasting for several minutes;
- Pain over shoulders, neck, left arm;
- Dizziness, shortness of breath;
- Sweating;
- Nausea;
- Unconsciousness.

If the artery is supplying a major portion of the heart, death may occur immediately. It does in 40 percent to 50 percent of the cases.

When the artery is sealed off, the heart muscle supplied by that artery ceases to function because of lack of oxygen and nutrients, and it dies. This damaged tissue area is referred to as *myocardial infarction. Myocardial* means heart muscle, and *infarction* means death to tissue.

Many factors have been identified that contribute to the quickening of the atherosclerosis process and cardiovascular disorders. They basically fall into two categories: those we cannot control and those we can control either by ourselves or with the assistance of a physician.

Factors We Cannot Control

1. *Heredity.* A history of cardiovascular diseases in your family means increased risk for the disease. A history usually means family members (parents, grandparents, brothers, sisters) have died from some cardiovascular disease before age sixty. Influencing factors may be an inherited genetic failure to deal effectively with blood fats. Some families have such a strong inherited genetic weakness that few males have lived past age forty.

2. *Sex.* Statistics reveal that cardiovascular disease is more prevalent in men than in women, especially before age forty-five. After age forty-five the difference lessens. This is probably due to the protective function of the female sex hormone, estrogen, in delaying the atherosclerosis process. The amount of estrogen after menopause is significantly reduced; thus its benefit is not as great for females after age forty-five.

3. *Age.* We know that as we grow older the chances of cardiovascular diseases increase. Sixty percent of deaths over age sixty-five are due to heart attacks but only 11 percent occur in persons aged fifteen to twenty-four.

A point to be emphasized is that even though you cannot control these three factors that are related to cardiovascular diseases, you can take two important steps related to them. First, if you have a family history of heart disease and have some of the other controlled factors, by all means emphasize controlling the factors you *can* control to compensate for any weakness in the areas you *can't* control.

Second, don't worry! You may say, "Oh, woe is me! My dad died at age forty-five of a heart attack, and so will I!" Don't accept that. You were created and wonderfully made by God despite any weaknesses or shortcomings you have. Cast your cares upon Him. You do your part and expect that God, who created you, will do His part. Worry can only hasten the problem. "For the thing I greatly feared has come upon me" (Job 3:25).

Factors We Can Control

Fortunately, research has been identifying factors related to cardiovascular diseases that we can control. They are related to lifestyle and make the greatest contribution toward reducing this disease. Many factors could be listed, but only the key ones will be mentioned here. They will be discussed further in later chapters.

1. *High blood pressure (hypertension).* It is estimated that more than thirty million Americans have high blood pressure. Approximately 37

percent of the blacks and 18 percent of the whites suffer from it. It usually begins in children, teen-agers, or young adults in their early twenties. A few new cases develop after age thirty. It is a silent disease, often with no symptoms. If left untreated with age, it greatly increases the risk of heart disease, stroke, and kidney failure.

Children are just as likely to suffer damage by hypertension as adults. In fact, the earlier in life the problem starts, the more severe the consequences. However, in nearly all cases, the risk can be greatly reduced by effectively controlling high blood pressure through a combination of diet, reduced salt intake, weight loss to an acceptable body composition, exercise, and, if necessary, medication.

2. *Smoking.* Smoking is estimated to cause 325,000 premature deaths each year due to lung cancer and heart disease. The risk of heart attack is much greater for the smoker than the nonsmoker.

3. *Obesity and excess weight.* As we will discuss in a later chapter, it is not so much your weight that is related to cardiovascular disease, as it is how much of your body weight is composed of fat. Excess body fat of twenty pounds or more triples your chances of heart attack.

4. *Physical inactivity and low fitness.* Lack of physical activity and low fitness are related to increased cardiovascular diseases. Studies have shown that persons engaged in active work that results in increased fitness enjoy reduced incidence of heart disease. Comparative studies of British bus drivers who sit versus ticket takers who walk, mail sorters who sit and sort mail versus those who walk and deliver the mail, and longshoremen who have heavy jobs versus those with office jobs favor the more active job for optimal health. Aerobics expert Dr. Kenneth Cooper has reported that his findings from the Institute for Aerobics Research reveal that the number one factor related to having a heart attack is low fitness as measured by a treadmill test. The second highest factor is obesity.

A recent study of 17,000 Harvard alumni revealed that those who regularly exercised at least three hours per week suffered 64 percent fewer heart attacks than those who did not exercise. And of those who did have heart attacks, 49 percent who do not have a history of physical activity die within four weeks, whereas only 17 percent of those who had a good history of physical activity die within four weeks.

5. *Elevated blood fats.* A number of blood fats essential for life are normally in the blood stream. These include cholesterol, phospholipids, triglycerides, and fatty acids. Research has shown that greater than acceptable fat levels in blood are related to atherosclerosis. Elevated blood lipids contribute to heart disease and seem to be related to lack of exercise, faulty diet, obesity, and heredity.

6. *Emotional stress*. Stress that causes tension within the body can lead to a number of physical ailments including heart disease. Persons under high emotional stress have been found to have elevated blood cholesterol levels, elevated blood pressure, and increased incidence of heart disease.

7. *Diabetes*. Diabetes is a disorder in which the body is unable to transfer sugar from the blood into the cell where it can be used for energy. As a result, sugar builds up in the blood. The primary cause of the disease is either a lack of insulin or a decreased sensitivity of the cell to insulin, since insulin is essential to carry sugar from the blood across the cell wall into the cell. Diabetes diagnosed in childhood is genetically related and usually requires medication to control. Diabetes that develops as an adult (adult onset diabetes) is usually related to lifestyle including obesity, lack of exercise, and a high sugar diet. Therefore, adult onset diabetes should be able to be prevented. This will be discussed more completely in a later chapter.

As in the case of hypertension, too often diabetes is left undetected and silently does its damage to the person over many years without the person's being aware of it. Diabetics have double the heart-disease problems of nondiabetics. The life expectancy of a thirty-five-year-old untreated diabetic is sixty-three years, compared to the normal seventy-six. Therefore, if individuals do not change their lifestyles and treat diabetes, thirteen years are subtracted from their life expectancy.

Why Exercise?

A program of regular physical exercise is critical because exercise can play a role in lowering the risk from six of the seven factors that contribute significantly to cardiovascular diseases. (Smoking is the only nonrelated exercise factor.) Regular exercise can benefit the cardiovascular system in various ways that have been demonstrated through research and through numerous personal testimonies.

A Test You Can Take

Evaluate your chances of having a heart attack by reading each section and recording your score.

1. *Heredity* (consider parents, grandparents,
   brothers, sisters)   Score _____
   a. No relative under 75 with heart disease   0
   b. One relative between 65 and 75 with heart
      disease   1
   c. Two relatives between 65 and 75 with heart
      disease   2

d. One or two relatives 55 to 65 with heart disease   4
e. One or two relatives under 55 with heart disease   6
f. Three or more relatives under 55 with heart
disease   8

2. *Age*   Score _____
   a. Less than 10   0
   b. 10–20   1
   c. 21–30   2
   d. 31–40   3
   e. 41–50   4
   f. 51–60   6
   g. 61 plus   8

3. *Sex*   Score _____
   a. Female under 40   0
   b. Female 40–50   1
   c. Female over 50   3
   d. Male under 50   3
   e. Male 50 plus   5

4. *Blood Pressure*★   Score _____
   a. Systolic under 100   0
   b. Systolic 100–120   1
   c. Systolic 121–135   2
   d. Systolic 136–150   3
   e. Systolic 151–165   4
   f. Systolic 166–180   6
   g. Systolic over 180   8

5. *Smoking*   Score _____
   a. Nonsmoker   0
   b. Cigar or pipe   2
   c. 10 or fewer cigarettes a day   2
   d. 10–20   "   "   "   4
   e. 21–30   "   "   "   6
   f. 31–40   "   "   "   8
   g. Over 40 "   "   "   10

6. *Obesity and Excess Weight*   Score _____
   a. Within 5 lbs normal weight   0
   b. 6–20 lbs over   1
   c. 21–35 lbs over   3
   d. 36–50 lbs over   5
   e. 51–80 lbs over   7
   f. More than 80 lbs over   10

7. *Exercise and Fitness*★★   Score _____
   Can jog 3 miles:

Men	*Women*	
Under 18 minutes	Under 21 minutes	0
18–21 minutes	21–24 minutes	1
21–24 minutes	24–28 minutes	2
24–28 minutes	28–32 minutes	4
28–32 minutes	32–36 minutes	6
32–36 minutes	36–40 minutes	8
36 plus minutes	40 plus minutes	10

8. *Cholesterol*★★★   Score _____
   a. Below 160   0
   b. 160–200   1
   c. 200–230   2
   d. 230–260   4
   e. 260–300   6
   f. 300 plus   8

9. *Emotional Stress*   Score _____
   a. I *always* feel relaxed, *nothing*
   ever bothers me.   0
   b. I occasionally get uptight.   2
   c. I get uptight several times per week.   4
   d. I get uptight usually once a day or more.   6
   e. I am usually in a hurry; there is just not
   enough time to get things done.
   People sometimes get in my way. To
   accomplish my goals, I often feel tense.   8

                                            Total Score _____

Risk Factor Score:
    6–13—well below average   30–36—above average
    14–22—below average   37–44—high level
    23–29—average   45 plus—very high

★If you don't know, score 2.

★★*Do not attempt this run* unless you are in good physical condition and have been cleared by a physician. Score 10 if you do not meet this criterion.

★★★If you don't know your cholesterol, score 4. If you emphasize a low-fat diet, then score 2.

This chart is only an estimate of risk factors and should not be considered an actual prediction of either having or not having a heart attack; however, if your risk is high, you should take steps to lower it.

7

Exercise

Our Story

A lifestyle of poor health habits is often developed in the teen-age years, but the results may not be felt until individuals reach their thirties, forties, or fifties. Fortunately, my wife, Donna, and I changed our lifestyle early and have been able to reap the benefits of that change.

Our story is not unlike that of most Americans. We were married before my sophomore year of college, when I was nineteen. I weighed 180 pounds and Donna 104 (I'm six feet one and Donna is five feet). I had always been active, participating in high school football, basketball, and baseball, and was all-conference in all three.

In college I continued to play football so I stayed in good (not excellent) physical condition. Football does not necessarily produce excellent cardiorespiratory fitnesss. My weight gradually climbed to 195 pounds by my senior year, but I still wore thirty-four-inch-waist slacks; therefore, the increasae in weight was primarily muscle resulting from weight training.

Upon graduation from college, I began graduate studies in exercise physiology, worked part-time in a physiology laboratory, assisted part-time in coaching a college football team, and was extremely busy for three years. My personal exercise program was significantly less than it was in college. I was still sports oriented and played an occasional game of racquetball, basketball, tennis, or golf. My weight went to 205 pounds, and my slacks size went to thirty-six—and that was tight.

During my third year of graduate studies, while I was conducting research on the benefits of exercise, I tested myself and found that the three years I had been participating only in recreational sports had been detrimental to my health. My body fat was up to 20.5 percent, time on the treadmill-graded exercise test was poor, and the ability of my cardio-respiratory system to deliver oxygen to my cells (aerobic capacity) was low. What I had been studying about the detrimental effects of lack of exercise on the body was happening to me. I knew I had to do something about it.

I changed my lifestyle in two respects. First, I cut back on snacks and desserts and ate more fruits and vegetables. Second, I began jogging, following the program described in chapter 8. Since I had a previous good fitness base, within a year my weight dropped back to 180 and my body fat to 13 percent. I was again able to wear slacks with a thirty-four-inch waist, my aerobic capacity increased to the good-to-excellent category, and I was jogging between twenty and twenty-five miles per week. I have followed this program for seventeen years, and I'm still at these fitness values. Thus, I have lost no health or fitness from age twenty-five to age forty.

Donna's history is quite a bit more dramatic. She had never been active in sports or exercise. In fact, she was poorly skilled in most sports and didn't enjoy them. Her weight gradually increased, after two children, to 117 pounds. Her clothes were size seven when we were married, but increased to size nine and even size eleven in some clothes.

About the same time I began my program, Donna began hers. Since she had never jogged before, she began by walking and pushing our daughter in the stroller. It took a year before she jogged her first mile without walking and two more years to jog three miles nonstop. However, by age twenty-eight, three years after she began, her weight had dropped to one hundred, she wore a size five and an occasional size three, and she had 16 percent body fat. She has maintained this for the past twelve years by jogging twenty to thirty miles per week.

In 1978 she became motivated to run a marathon and increased her mileage to forty to fifty miles per week and successfully completed the twenty-six-mile course. During this time, she increased her food intake but she still dropped to ninety-seven pounds because of the calories burned by the additional jogging.

One of the greatest enjoyments of our marriage has been jogging together. We often jog three to five miles at a time. In the hustle and bustle of life, these times together have been quality time when we discuss the events of the day and our family. We enjoy the beauty of the outdoors, and we significantly contribute to ourselves and each other as we take care of our bodies and keep them healthy. On our wedding anniversary we jog the number of years we have been married. In 1984 that meant twenty-two miles!

As I mentioned earlier, Donna had never been athletically inclined. One day, before she had started her jogging program, we went water-skiing with some friends. It was Donna's first attempt. She tried several times but could not get out of the water. The next day she was extremely sore. Some thirteen years later, after she had developed a high level of fitness from jogging and muscle-development exercise, she again attempted to water-ski. This time she did it very easily, skied for a good part of the day, and had no soreness the next day. It pays to build a basis of fitness since it makes everything else easier.

Am I Too Old to Exercise—Especially to Jog?

One of the major excuses people use not to exercise is, "I'm too old for that." Nonsense! If you're alive and breathing, you're not too old to exercise. You may or may not be able to jog, but there is some form of exercise you can do. The older you get, the more exercise you need. In fact, many people haven't started to exercise until their fifties or sixties.

Patricia Ryan, R.N., who had previously not engaged in any exercise, began walking for exercise at age fifty-seven. By age sixty she had progressed to walking/jogging three miles a day. Her newfound fitness added vigor, and her enthusiasm for jogging increased to the extent that she stopped walking and began jogging and increased her mileage to four and five miles per day. At age sixty-two she ran her first race of ten kilometers (6.2 miles) and won her age division. She gradually ran longer races (fifteen and twenty-five kilometers) until, at age sixty-four, she entered and completed her first marathon (twenty-six miles). She retired at age sixty-five from the Student Health Clinic at Oral Roberts University (ORU) and took a five-year hitch as a Christian missionary nurse in a hospital in Israel. Her optimal health that resulted from her exercise program has enabled her to be a minister of the gospel when others her age are retiring and sitting at home.

Richard Patty retired at age sixty-one and asked himself the questions, Can a sixty-one-year-old be as fit as a thirty-year-old in excellent condition? and Would being as fit as a thirty-year-old in excellent condition be worth the time, effort, and money required? To answer these questions Richard started a fitness program. It took a year before he could jog one mile without stopping. In one more year he made additional progress and spent about ten hours per week on the program. During the third year he decided to "go for it." He enrolled in an adult fitness class and devoted almost twenty hours per week to get his body in the shape he desired. During that year, he walked/jogged 1,525 miles, cycled 1,600 miles, and swam 105 miles. He then returned to his physician for a complete physical exam. The cardiologist said that the EKG stress test showed Richard had, in fact, achieved the shape of an excellently conditioned thirty-year-old. The doctor knew of no charts for Richard's age that included such a high level of fitness. He has eased up on his development program and follows a maintenance program today, but he has answered his initial two questions with a resounding yes.

At age fifty, a Tulsa bank vice president weighed 205 pounds and had several lifestyle habits conducive to bad health. His doctor said he was living too high on the hog and he should make some changes. By age fifty-two, in just two years, he was jogging sixty miles per week (ten miles, six days a week), he was down to 170 pounds, and he had jogged a twenty-six-mile marathon in three hours and thirty-seven minutes. When he began, he doubted he could do it, but now he finds it exhilarating. He jogs late in the afternoon and reflects on what occurred that day at the bank, plans his agenda for the next day, mentally writes letters, and occasionally listens to tapes.

I could go on and on with testimonials on exercise and what it has done for people: Larry Lewis who was still jogging at 103, Mrs. Lamb who is still jogging at 90, and Johnny Kelly who in his late seventies has run the twenty-six-mile Boston Marathon for fifty years in a row. In fact, in the 1981 Boston Marathon, seventy-seven runners were over age 65.

Health Benefits from Regular Physical Exercise

The benefits of exercise upon the body depend upon the type of exercise done, the intensity and duration of the exercise, the number of times the exercise was done per week, and the weeks, months, and even years the exercise was continued. The specifics of exercise will be discussed in the next two chapters. If you engage in a comprehensive exercise program as outlined in the rest of the book, you can expect the following beneficial results.

1. *Heart.* The resting heart rate will decrease. If your resting heart rate is more than 60, it will drop anywhere from 10 to 25 beats per minute. Before Donna began her jogging program, her resting heart rate was 80 beats per minute. Now it is 55. When it beat at 80, her heart was beating 115,200 times per day, 806,400 times per week, and 41,932,800 times per year. Now with her heart rate at 55, her heart is beating 79,200 times per day, 554,400 times per week, and 28,828,800 times per year. Therefore, in one year her heart beat 13,104,000 fewer times than it did before. Her heart doesn't have to work as hard to accomplish the same work. It rests more and will last much longer. I'm all for that. My resting heart rate is 48.

When you exercise, the better your fitness, the slower your heart will beat. Recently I jogged three miles in twenty-four minutes with an ORU cross-country runner. After the run my pulse was 150 but the other runner's was only 110. My heart had a good workout, but the runner's heart was in such great shape that it was hardly working to accomplish the same task. This is because a conditioning program will strengthen the heart muscle, enabling it to pump more blood per contraction. Also, the maximum amount of blood it can pump per minute can be approximately thirty quarts compared to an unconditioned person's eight to twelve quarts. More blood will reach the heart muscle via the coronary arteries; therefore, the heart will fatigue less easily and have greater resistance to heart attack.

2. *Blood vessels.* The blood vessels will have greater elasticity and distensibility (ability to expand or stretch) which will help lower blood pressure. There will be less atherosclerosis, and more capillaries will function to deliver more oxygen to cells, thus enabling all the body's cells to function better. Also, the blood vessels will increase their ability to open (vasodilate) and close (vasoconstrict) and deliver the blood to where the need is greatest at any given time.

3. *Blood.* Regular exercise can increase the oxygen-carrying capacity of the blood by increasing the hemoglobin in the blood. It can also lower blood lipids that contribute to atherosclerosis: cholesterol, triglycerides, and low-density lipoproteins (LDL). Recent research has discovered that high-density lipoproteins (HDL) seem to inhibit the atherosclerosis process, and long-duration exercise appears to increase this lipid in the blood.

4. *Pulmonary system.* Regular exercise improves the functioning of the pulmonary system in several ways. The lungs will allow more oxygen to be diffused into the blood. When you begin to exercise regularly, your lungs will favorably adapt to the demand and will function more efficiently. You will become less winded as you walk or engage in any physical activity. You can take in far greater amounts of oxygen when needed.

5. *Lymphatic circulation.* The lymphatic system is poorly understood by most people, but it is extremely important. Its function is to assist in the removal of wastes and toxic substances from the cells and carry them to the blood stream where the kidneys can rid the body of them. The body cells must be in a nontoxic environment to function properly; therefore, there is a constant need to void the wastes since cells are constantly working and giving off wastes. When you exercise, your body's movements and the contractions of your muscles help significantly to increase the lymphatic circulation thereby ridding the cells of their waste products. Every cell in the body can function more effectively, can resist disease better, is in a better environment, and is less likely to deteriorate. This is one big bonus of daily exercise.

6. *Skeletal muscles.* While some of the benefits of exercise often go un-noticed, skeletal-muscle changes are often more visible. The muscles will be stronger and less likely to develop soreness. If men engage in heavy weight training, their muscles will get larger; however, this won't occur in women. The muscles can become more flexible and less likely to tear. One of the greatest benefits can be a resistance to the nagging problem of back pain.

7. *Weight and fat control.* Too many people think all these benefits are desirable, but their only real concern is, Will exercise help me lose weight? The answer is a definite yes! We will discuss this more thoroughly in chapters 14 and 15. Losing fat through exercise is a gradual process but will pay fantastic dividends if you don't give up when you don't see immediate results.

8. *Bones.* Recent studies reveal that regular exercise also helps to strengthen bones. Calcium deposition in the bones is increased, resulting in stronger bones and less *osteoporosis* (increased porosity of bones). Hip fractures in women over age sixty-five cost $6 billion a year, and many women die within a year of the injury. This statistic could be dramatically improved if all people exercised. Many persons take calcium pills to strengthen their bones. However, calcium alone, without the stimulus of exercise, will not strengthen them.

9. *General health.* The specific benefits to the various organs and systems of your body all work together to greatly improve your overall general health. You feel better, suffer less fatigue, have more energy to perform your daily tasks, resist disease better, meet emergencies better, and have greater vitality. Numerous studies show that physically fit persons are sick less often, see their doctor less, are hospitalized less, and spend less on medical care than persons who are not physically fit.

A study from the Massachusetts General Hospital reported that 86 percent of hospitalizations probably could have been prevented if patients had followed a healthful lifestyle. Separate studies done on employees of Northern Natural Gas, Allen Bradley Co., New York State Department of Education and Civil Services, NASA, and Purdue University reported less sickness, better health, better job performance, and fewer health insurance claims among employees who were physically fit. Businessess are beginning to realize that they can't afford to hire unfit employees. In the last ten years more than three hundred companies have started fitness programs for their employees.

10. *Mental and emotional health.* A regular exercise program has substantial psychological benefits. You will feel less tension, be able to relax more, experience less depression, and have a better attitude toward work and life in general.

11. *Personal appearance.* A regular exercise program can greatly improve your personal appearance. Reduced body weight, less body fat, better muscle tone, return of your natural body curves, and delay in the aging process all contribute to better appearance. This can produce an enhanced self-concept and body image. Many women have said to Donna, "You're so lucky to be tiny." *It's not luck.* It's the result of a lifestyle.

Steps You Could Take

You can receive these benefits as easily as anyone else. It is up to you. Do you really want to look great, feel great, have energy and strength to be active all day, get into clothes two sizes smaller, and "run and not be weary"? If you really want to live a longer life of increased vigor and optimal health, follow the lifestyle described in this book and you will.

8

Aerobics for Health

A frequent question is, If exercise is beneficial, what kind of exercises should I do? Much misinformation is contained in the answers. Different exercises produce different results.

I knew a marathon runner who could run twenty-six miles in under three hours, and he faithfully ran fifty to sixty miles every week. He had great fitness in his heart, lungs, and legs, but his upper body was weak. He did no exercises for his arms, shoulders, abdomen, and back. He could do no pull-ups, about ten pushups, and barely twenty situps. I recommended that he add upper-body, back, and abdominal exercises to his jogging to develop total fitness. Unfortunately, he ignored the advice, claiming that jogging was the total exercise. Predictably, he developed a back problem severe enough to curtail his jogging for six months.

He learned that exercises are specific to various systems of the body and that jogging will not result in total body fitness. During his rehabilitation his body responded well to a back exercise program, and now he is jogging fifty miles per week again. But he also does fifty situps, twenty-five pushups, and several back exercises every day.

Types of Exercise

What we need to understand is the critical concept of *specificity of training*. This concept states that certain exercises will give specific benefits to the body but no single exercise will benefit all aspects of the body. Unfortunately, many persons claim one exercise does it all. If you look in any bookstore or go to many health spas, you see the promoters of such a misunderstanding.

There are basically three general categories of exercises, and each has specific application for benefiting different parts of the body.

1. *Muscle-development exercises.* The primary purpose of muscle-development exercises is to develop the muscles of the body that control movement. These exercises include chiefly weight training, isometrics, and calisthenics. They are vital in developing strength, flexibility, muscle tone, and body contours, in maintaining posture, and in preventing back pain. They are an essential and important part of a total exercise program. These will be discussed in chapters 10 and 11.
2. *Aerobic exercises.* The primary purpose of aerobic exercises is to develop the cardiorespiratory system and to assist in controlling body weight by decreasing the total amount of body fat. They are important in strengthening the heart and related organs and are beneficial in preventing heart disease. Aerobic exercises are an absolute part of any total exercise program. They include walking, jogging, cycling, and swimming. Guidelines for aerobic exercises will be described later in this chapter and in chapter 9.
3. *Anaerobic exercises.* The primary function of an anaerobic exercise is to develop speed, quickness, agility, balance, and similar characteristics. They include sprinting, undergoing high-intensity interval training, running quickly up hills or stairs, doing agility drills used in sports activities, swimming underwater, and working through other high-intensity activities of short duration. Anaerobic exercises are especially important for athletes but are not a normal part of a regular adult total exercise program. In fact, they can be damaging to the health of an adult and can be fatal.

Of the three types of exercise, *muscle-development* and *aerobic exercises* are the core of a good exercise program.

Why Aerobics?

To understand aerobics and why aerobic exercises are critical for health, we must better understand our constant need for oxygen. We can live only where oxygen is present. Since we cannot absorb oxygen into our cells directly through our skin, we must inhale it from the air into our lungs. There the oxygen diffuses into the blood stream, is picked up by the iron portion of the hemoglobin of the red blood cell, and is transported through the blood stream by the pumping action of the heart. It eventually diffuses out of the blood stream and goes to a cell where it combines with fats or carbohydrates to give energy. This energy is used by the cell to contract the muscles, cause cell reproduction, repair cells, cause growth of cells and secretion of hormones, or bring about a multitude of other cellular functions. Without oxygen, the cells would not have the energy to perform their work.

For the cells to function at rest, approximately two hundred to three hundred milliliters of oxygen must be delivered to the cells per minute. When you eat a meal, your oxygen need increases to about four hundred milliliters per minute because more blood is sent to your stomach. As you walk, jog, swim, or cycle, your muscles are contracting more and demanding more energy; therefore more oxygen must be delivered to your cells. Your body makes adjustments by breathing harder, your heart beats faster and pumps more blood, and so on.

Persons who are fit have a great capacity to adjust to the increased demand of the cells for oxygen, up to as high as six thousand milliliters of oxygen per minute. Poorly fit persons' hearts, lungs, and other systems are not as healthy and cannot adjust to high demands. They may be able to deliver only one thousand milliliters of oxygen to the cells per minute.

When you are exercising at a low intensity and the need for oxygen is being met by body adjustments, that exercise is called an *aerobic* (with oxygen) exercise. The oxygen needed to meet the energy demand of the cells for the exercise is being supplied, and no waste products other than carbon dioxide are being produced.

On the other hand, when you are exercising at a high intensity and the need for oxygen is not being met by body adjustments, that exercise is called an *anaerobic* (without oxygen) exercise. The immense energy needed by the cells for the exercise is not supplied by sufficient oxygen intake, and waste products, primarily lactic acid, are produced. This will lead to pain and exhaustion. Anaerobic exercises usually last less than five minutes due to the build-up of pain-producing waste products.

The heart in anaerobic exercise is working as hard as it can, but it can't meet the demand. If the heart is not in good condition, this demand can have a damaging effect and can actually precipitate a heart attack. Therefore, anaerobic exercises are not for poorly conditioned individuals but rather for the young athlete and the highly fit adult.

The Heart-rate Criterion

How do you determine whether an exercise is aerobic or anaerobic? Here's a practical guideline. If you are unable to talk while doing the exercise (the Talk Test), it is probably anaerobic and you should ease up. If while walking, jogging, or cycling with a friend, you can carry on a continual conversation, the exercise intensity is probably aerobic.

A better, more accurate, and scientific guideline in determining if the exercise is aerobic is to measure your heart rate. Since the heart speeds up in response to the cells' need for oxygen, it reflects the activity in the cells. As the cells demand more oxygen, the heart will beat faster until it reaches its maximum rate. The maximum varies according to age and sex. If there is no underlying heart disease or the person is not on medication, Table 8.1 predicts maximal heart rate.

TABLE 8.1
Predicted Maximal Heart Rate
According to Age and Sex

AGE	MEN	WOMEN
20	200	205
25	195	200
30	190	195
35	185	190
40	180	185
45	175	180
50	170	175
55	166	170
60	163	165
65+	160	160

*Maximum heart rate decreases slightly after age 65.

For most persons, the body can meet the oxygen demand of the cells up to the point that the heart rate reaches 85 percent of its maximum. Beyond 85 percent, the body begins to switch to anaerobic metabolism. Therefore, the *first guideline* in an aerobic exercise program is that the *heart rate should not exceed 85 percent of your age-adjusted maximum*.

The *second guideline* that must be followed relates to the exercise principle called *overload*. For the heart to become stronger, for the lungs to increase their efficiency, and the entire cardiovascular system to achieve optimal health and fitness, they must work harder than they are accustomed to working. A demand must be placed upon them. The intensity for the minimal stimulus required to cause a benefit to this system is approximately 65 percent of an individual's maximal heart rate. Therefore, the second guideline for an aerobic exercise program is that *the heart rate should equal or exceed 65 percent of your age-adjusted maximum*.

Guidelines one and two can be combined in the following table.

Medical Clearance

Since an aerobic exercise program is based upon exercise that will cause the heart to beat at 65 percent to 85 percent of its maximum, such a program has two prerequisites. The first is that you must *consult your physician*, preferably one who believes in and follows a regular exercise program. What the physician's evaluation involves will vary. If you are

TABLE 8.2
Minimum and Maximum
Aerobic Exercise Heart-rate Range
According to Age and Sex

AGE	WOMEN'S EXERCISE HEART-RATE RANGE			MEN'S EXERCISE HEART-RATE RANGE		
	MINIMUM 65%	MIDRANGE 75%	MAXIMUM 85%	MINIMUM 65%	MIDRANGE 75%	MAXIMUM 85%
20	135	155	175	130	150	170
25	132	152	171	127	147	166
30	128	148	167	123	143	162
35	125	145	162	120	140	157
40	122	142	158	117	137	153
45	119	139	154	114	134	149
50	116	136	150	111	131	145
55	112	132	145	108	128	141
60	109	129	141	106	126	139
65+	105	125	136	105	125	136

low risk and below age thirty-five to forty, a minimal evaluation is required. However, if you are high risk or older than thirty-five, a resting and exercise electrocardiogram should be included in the evaluation. Discuss the exercises recommended in this chapter with your physician and receive medical clearance before you begin to exercise.

Second, you need to know how to *count your own heart rate*. It would be easier to measure the time it takes to walk or jog a selected distance, but we want the best program using the knowledge God has given us. By counting your heart rate this is a specific program for you. Therefore, while it may involve a little more knowledge on your part, the benefits will be greater.

You *can* learn to count your own heart rate. It doesn't take a doctor or a nurse. Two locations can be used. One is the brachial artery in your wrist (thumb side of wrist); the other is the carotid artery in the neck (adjacent to the voice box). Find your pulse by placing your fingers (not your thumb) gently over the artery, and count the pulsations. Get some assistance if necessary. (Everybody knows at least one nurse.) Then practice, practice, practice! You must be accurate. Count your pulse for six seconds using a second hand on a clock or watch and add a zero. If you count ten in six seconds, your heart rate is one hundred per minute. If you count seven in six seconds, your heart rate is seventy. Learn to accurately count your heart rate before you begin your exercise program.

What Should My Aerobic Exercise Goal Be?

Guidelines one and two gave the criteria for the intensity of the exercise (65 percent to 85 percent of your maximal heart rate). Now, how many minutes do you perform the exercise and how many days per week? Let me describe here what the goal should be, and in the next section I will provide a progressive program that will lead you to that goal.

Research has demonstrated that to have excellent cardiovascular fitness and to be in optimal health, you should engage in an aerobic exercise program *a minimum of three but preferably five days per week*, the intensity should be 65 percent to 85 percent of your maximum, and the duration should be *thirty to sixty minutes*. Once you get to a level of fitness where you can do this three to five days per week without producing muscle soreness or fatigue, you will probably be in excellent cardiovascular condition.

| | DURATION (MINUTES) | |
INTENSITY	MINIMAL	OPTIMAL
65%	30	60
75%	20	45
85%	10	30

The intensity and duration variations should be selected in combination with each other. If the intensity is high, the duration can be shorter. However, the same benefit to the body can be realized if the intensity is low and the duration longer.

TABLE 8.3 Progression Rate 1*

WEEK	HEART-RATE INTENSITY (%)	DURATION IN MINUTES
1	65	15
2	65	25
3	65	35
4	65–75	40
5	65–75	45
6	75	45
7	75–85	30–35
8	75–85	30–40
9th and thereafter (85–30, 75–45, 65–60)		

*Progression rate 1 is for persons under age 25 who are not overweight and have participated in some kind of exercise program within the past 2 years. Beginning with the ninth week they can choose their exercise intensity-duration of either 85% for 30 minutes, 75% for 45 minutes, or 65% for 60 minutes.

The same approximate benefits to the body will be achieved from any of these three combinations. For example, on one day of the week you may have more time to exercise so you walk/jog sixty minutes at 65 percent intensity. The next day your time for exercise is limited so you walk/jog thirty minutes at 85 percent intensity. You choose the combination at which you desire to exercise. Persons over age sixty should probably avoid the 85 percent intensity. However, if you are in excellent condition and your body tolerates the 85 percent intensity, then that level is acceptable.

For those who are highly motivated and desire to go beyond the above recommendations, feel free to do so. If you want to go on to marathon running or road races, that's great. These recommendations will produce excellent fitness, but the body is capable of superior fitness. So, have at it. (See the appendix for a marathon training schedule.)

However, if you can faithfully meet the goal listed above, you will reach fitness necessary for optimal health. Beyond that, the aerobics program becomes more of a hobby than a basic program for your personal health and fitness. Also, going beyond can result in an occasional orthopedic problem. Be careful.

Where Do I Start?

A major reason people don't continue their exercise program is that they are highly motivated and begin with too intense a program. Too fast a start leads to muscle pain, joint pain, or other complications that cause

TABLE 8.4 Progression Rate 2*

WEEK	HEART-RATE INTENSITY (%)	DURATION IN MINUTES
1	65	10
2	65	15
3	65	20
4	65–75	25
5	65–75	30
6	65–75	35
7	65–75	40
8	65–75	45
9	75	45
10	75–85	30
11	75–85	30–35
12	75–85	30–40
13th week and thereafter (85–30, 75–45, 65–60)		

*Progression rate 2 is for persons ages 25–45 but also should be followed by persons under age 25 who are 15 to 25 pounds overweight or who haven't exercised within the past 2 years.

discouragement and lead to ending the exercise program. If you have not engaged in a regular exercise program for a year or more and if you have excess body fat, you need to begin gradually and progress slowly. *Don't start out at the higher intensity and optimal duration just outlined!*

Some time ago a sixty-one-year-old woman who was twenty-five pounds overweight and considerably out of shape attended one of my seminars on fitness. She decided she would start her own fitness program. She didn't, however, pay full attention to the advice on gradual progression, and she started out attempting to walk/jog thirty minutes at 85 percent of her maximum heart rate (for her, a heart rate of 141). After

TABLE 8.5
Progression Rate 3*

WEEK	HEART-RATE INTENSITY (%)	DURATION IN MINUTES
1	65	10
2	65	15
3	65	20
4	65	25
5	65	30
6	65	35
7	65	40
8	65	45
9	65–75	35
10	65–75	40
11	75	35
12	75	40
13	75	45
14	75–85	30
15	75–85	30–35
16	75–85	30–40
17th week and thereafter (85–30, 75–45, 65–60)		

*Progression rate 3 is for persons ages 45–60 but also for persons under age 45 who are 25 to 35 pounds overweight.

fifteen minutes she quit because of exhaustion, went home, and was in bed for the rest of the day. She decided that exercise was not for her.

When I became aware of her plight, I reviewed with her the need to begin gradually. Because she was in poor shape, overweight, and over sixty years of age, I recommended a gradual progression listed in Progression Rate 4. Now, one year later, she is walking sixty minutes at 125 beats per minute (75 percent of her maximum) with no ill effects. She has significantly improved her fitness and has lost fifteen of her twenty-five excess pounds.

So that you may start at the appropriate intensity and duration, Tables 8.3 through 8.6 list four different progression rates on the basis of age, weight, and exercise history for a person who has been medically cleared for exercise and has no cardiovascular problems. All progression rates are based upon exercising four to six days per week. Since these charts are estimates, you may progress more quickly if it is too easy or more slowly if you have difficulty keeping up with the progression.

TABLE 8.6
Progression Rate 4*

WEEK	HEART-RATE INTENSITY (%)	DURATION IN MINUTES
1	65	10
2	65	15
3	65	15
4	65	20
5	65	25
6	65	25
7	65	30
8	65	35
9	65	35
10	65	40
11	65	45
12	65–75	35
13	65–75	35
14	65–75	40
15	65–75	45
16	75	35
17	75	40
18	75	40
19	75	45
20	75–85	30
21	75–85	30–35
22	75–85	30–45
23rd week and thereafter (85–30, 75–45, 65–60)		

*Progression rate 4 is for persons over age 60 but also should be followed for persons under age 60 who are 35 to 45 pounds overweight. If a person is more than 45 pounds overweight, regardless of age, see the progression recommended in chapter 15.

The progression rates given are only guidelines and not absolutes. It cannot be predicted exactly how everybody will respond. The progression may be either speeded up or slowed down, but it is better to progress too slow than too fast. You don't run into problems with a slow progress, but you may with too fast a progression. It may take you a few weeks longer to arrive at your goal, but you'll get there just the same—all in one piece. And remember—this is a lifestyle; something you are going to do the rest of your life. Take your time and enjoy it along the way.

Additional Guidelines

I don't accept the idea of "no pain—no gain." Many persons, especially athletically inclined macho types, believe it has to hurt if you're going to get any benefit from any exercise. While you may experience greater gains faster from a program of high intensity that causes some discomfort or pain, this belief has several problems associated with it:

- It should be used only by a highly fit young person.
- The potential harmful effects far outweigh the benefits.
- It may cause irreparable damage that may prevent a future exercise program.
- Many persons won't put up with the pain and will not engage in an exercise program at all if too much discomfort is associated with it.

The principle we are emphasizing for a lifestyle of lifelong exercise is "train—don't strain." Become involved in an aerobic exercise program with the appropriate progression that will result in gradual benefits without any harmful side effects to your body or mind.

The following guidelines are given to evaluate whether your intensity and/or duration may be too great.

1. Five minutes after you finish your aerobic exercise, your heart rate should be below 120 if you were exercising at a heart rate above 150; below 110 if you were exercising at a heart rate in the 140s; below 105 if you were exercising at a heart rate in the 130s; and below 100 for all other persons.
2. After showering following your workout, you should feel refreshed and invigorated, not tired or exhausted.
3. If your muscles or joints bother you more than one day after your workout, you need to ease up.

Steps You Could Take

1. Look up on the chart (see Table 8.1) and record your predicted maximal heart rate.

2. What is your aerobic exercise heart-rate range?
(Example [see Table 8.2]. If predicted maximum heart rate is 200, then the 65% aerobic exercise heart rate would be 130.)

65% _____
75% _____
85% _____

3. Learn how to accurately count your heart rate.

4. Your goal for the future should be to exercise by walking, jogging, swimming, or cycling three to five days per week for sixty minutes at 65 percent, or forty-five minutes at 75 percent, or thirty minutes at 85 percent.

5. Select the appropriate progression rate (from Table 8.3, 8.4, 8.5, or 8.6) and fill out the chart showing your exercise plan and the number of weeks it will take to reach your goal. Select the particular activity after you read chapter 9 (after 9 weeks develop your own chart).

WEEK	INTENSITY (65%, 75%, or 85%)	HEART RATE	DURATION	ACTIVITY
Ex.	65%	130	15 min.	walk/jog M-W-F cycle Tu-Th
1				
2				
3				
4				
5				
6				
7				
8				
9				
etc.				

6. Fill in the record below to keep a log of your daily aerobic exercise program (after 4 weeks develop your own chart).

WEEK	DAY	ACTIVITY	HR[a]	Duration[b]	Distance[c]
	M	Walk	135	10	.5 mile
	Tu	Stat. Cycle	126	10	
Example	W	Walk	130	12	.6 mile
	Thu	Stat. Cycle	120	12	
	Sat	Walk	138	10	.5 mile
1					
2					
3					

4

_____ _____ _____ _____ _____
_____ _____ _____ _____ _____
_____ _____ _____ _____ _____
_____ _____ _____ _____ _____
_____ _____ _____ _____ _____
_____ _____ _____ _____ _____

[a] The heart rate will usually not be exactly at the planned intensity; if the HR is within 5–10 beats above or below, that is acceptable.

[b] The duration also may be longer if exercise is easy.

[c] Distance recording is optional, but it can be motivational to see you are going farther as weeks go by.

9

The "Big Three" Aerobic Exercises

Which Form of Aerobic Exercise Is Best?

In the previous chapter we described the guidelines for a good aerobic exercise program. Now we need to look at which forms of exercise will best meet these guidelines.

The basic guideline is that any physical activity that causes the heart to beat between 65 percent and 85 percent of its maximum and can maintain that heart rate for an appropriate duration will improve the functioning of the cardiorespiratory system. The aerobic activities that are considered to be the "big three" for developing the cardiorespiratory system are (1) walking/jogging, (2) cycling, and (3) swimming.

These forms of exercise place the most consistent overload upon the cardiorespiratory system because they are continuous and not intermittent; they can be aerobic and not anaerobic. Two excellent forms of walking/jogging are jumping on a trampoline and exercising to music. Cross-country skiing is also an outstanding aerobic activity but is not included here because it is not practical for many people.

Most sports, such as tennis, basketball, and racquetball, are intermittent. That is, they involve bursts of intense movement that are or border upon being an anaerobic activity, followed by periods of standing, walking, or resting between bouts. When an excess overload greater than 85 percent of the maximum heart rate is placed upon the cardiorespiratory system for a short time, usually the duration is too short to cause a benefit. This is followed by a period of low intensity where the intensity is less than 65 percent of the maximum and therefore is of little benefit to the body.

Any one of the big three will result in a comparable benefit to the cardiorespiratory system. Your selection should be based upon practical considerations. The following sections list some strengths and weaknesses of each activity.

Swimming

By swimming, we mean lap swimming, not playing in the water. Normally this means the crawl stroke, breast stroke, back stroke, or a combination of the three.

Strengths
1. In addition to its benefits to the cardiovascular system, it will develop upper-body strength.
2. It does not produce wear and tear on the joints.
3. People can swim with sprained ankles or injured knees. Even persons with handicapping conditions can swim. I have seen tremendous benefits to paraplegics and other physically limited persons who have used swimming both for therapy and for fitness.

Weaknesses
1. An individual must be a skilled swimmer capable of swimming the appropriate duration without stopping before benefits result. If a person is not a skilled swimmer, swimming is more anaerobic than aerobic.
2. A pool is required to swim in.
3. Monitoring the heart rate is difficult. (The heart rate while swimming should 5 to 10 beats fewer than the charts say. For example, if you jog at a heart rate of 140, then swim at a heart rate of 130 to 135.)
4. Less subcutaneous fat is lost than when jogging.
5. Swimming does little to exercise the legs.

Cycling

Cycling can be either indoor stationary cycling or cycling outdoors. Both provide identical physiological benefits, but each has somewhat different considerations.

Indoor Stationary Cycling
Strengths
1. In addition to its benefits to the cardiorespiratory system, it will develop leg strength.
2. It does not produce wear and tear on the joints.
3. It does not require skill.
4. It can be done in the home regardless of weather or time of day.

5. It generally does not produce injuries.
6. It can be done while watching TV or listening to radio or tapes.
7. Heart rate can be easily monitored.

Weaknesses
1. A good stationary cycle must be purchased, a minimum of $100 to $150.
2. A place in the home is required to store it.

Outdoor Cycling

Strengths
1. Same as 1 and 2 of indoor cycling.
2. Riding a cycle through beautiful neighborhoods and parks is enjoyable.

Weaknesses
1. A good cycle must be purchased, which may cost a minimum of $100 to $150.
2. It can be dangerous if there is no safe place to ride.
3. Some balance is required.
4. It does little to exercise the upper body.

Walking/Jogging

The walking/jogging category includes a number of activities you do while on your feet. These include walking alone, walking combined with some jogging, jogging alone, jumping on a trampoline, or exercising to music.

Walking/Jogging

Strengths
1. This is a minimal cost activity; the only equipment is a pair of good jogging shoes.
2. It is convenient. Walking/jogging can be done almost anywhere.
3. It can be social activity because conversation with another person is possible while exercising.
4. No skill is involved.

Weakness
1. It can cause joint problems if individuals jog on a hard surface, do not follow proper progression, or do not have good shoes.

Many people erroneously feel that walking is not sufficiently vigorous to produce benefits and that jogging is better. For some people this is true, but for the vast majority of adults much benefit can be derived from a walking program. The factor that determines whether you should walk or jog (assuming you have no joint problems) is your heart rate. If your heart rate is 65 percent to 85 percent of your maximum when you walk, then you should walk and not jog.

If your heart rate is well below 65 percent when you walk fast, then you will need to increase your energy demand by jogging. This will increase your heart rate above the minimum of 65 percent. Most persons start out their exercise program walking and their heart rate is in the 65 percent to 85 percent range. As your fitness increases, you will begin to alternate walking and jogging to keep your heart rate in the aerobic exercise range. Or you may walk fast with weights in each hand that will also elevate heart rate.

Myron Peace, who directed and helped establish the aerobics program at Oral Roberts University in the early 1970s, used the term *jog-walk* to describe the fast walking/slow jogging pace that persons go through when gradually switching from all walking to all jogging. In time, your heart muscle will be in such good shape that you will need to jog for the entire duration to keep your heart rate in the 65 percent to 85 percent range.

Jumping on Minitramps

Within the past five years a tremendous interest has developed in jumping on minitramps as a form of aerobic exercise. Part of the interest has been spurred by companies that have distributors all across the country. Many well-meaning zealots who lack exercise physiology knowledge have made various outlandish claims, such as "Five minutes of jumping is equivalent to a three-mile jog." Unfortunately, that is not true. But if you follow the guidelines previously given (65 percent to 85 percent maximum intensity for the appropriate duration), then the minitramps have definite aerobic value to the cardiorespiratory system.

Strengths
1. It is convenient because it can be done in the home regardless of time of day or weather conditions.
2. No skill is involved.
3. Because of the "give" of the surface, there is little or no joint trauma.
4. It can be done while watching TV or listening to the radio or tapes.

Weaknesses
1. A good minitramp must be purchased. While you can purchase one for less than $60, if it is used regularly, it won't last long. You probably need to pay $75 to $125 for a quality minitramp.
2. A place is needed for the minitramp. (However, some companies manufacture a minitramp that is like a big footstool with a removable cushion.)
3. Some balance and equilibrium are required.

Aerobics to Music

Aerobic Dance, founded by Jackie Sorenson, and Rhythmic Aerobics, founded by Nancy Kabriel, are two forms of aerobic exercise in which various movements are performed to music. These activities are especially popular with women and are taught in schools, YMCAs, YWCAs, health clubs, business, and industry. The activities are choreographed and set to music with low-, medium-, and high-intensity routines available. In fact, aerobic exercise to music has become so popular that when many people hear the term *aerobics*, they think of dance. Recently Nancy Kabriel has added "Devotion to Motion" in which exercises are performed to Christian music. Laura Rhodes has developed "Worship in Action" which was recently incorporated into "Creative Aerobics" by Sally Schollmeier. (For anyone interested in more information, write or call: Nancy Kabriel, Rhythmic Aerobics Inc., 8332 East 73rd St. South, Woodland Point Office, Suite 100, Tulsa, OK 74133; Sally Schollmeier, Instructor in Health Fitness, Oral Roberts University, Tulsa, OK 74171.)

Strengths
1. The music and variety of movements can be more enjoyable than performing just one activity (such as cycling) for the entire workout.
2. The exercises are often done in a group taught by a specialist so there is social interaction.
3. The variety of exercises has the potential of developing more of the body than just the cardiorespiratory system.

Weaknesses
1. Often the classes are taught in a location where the participants exercise on a hard surface. Extended exercise on a hard surface can lead to joint problems and shin splints.
2. If the class is taught one or two days per week and the person doesn't exercise at least three to five days per week, the benefit to the body will be negligible.
3. It can be similar to intermittent work and has the potential of causing the heart rate to exceed 85 percent during intense times and going below 65 percent during resting times if not monitored carefully.

Which Form of Aerobic Exercise Should I Do?

Since all three forms of aerobic exercises have the potential of producing comparable benefits, you should evaluate your personal situation and review the strengths and weaknesses of each of the activities. Donna's basic aerobics program involves jogging five or six days per week, usually twenty-five to thirty miles per week, fifty-two weeks of the year.

My personal program is basically jogging, but I mix in some swimming and cycling. I will jog three to four days per week, usually swim two days per week, and occasionally cycle instead of jog. I prefer the variety in order to prevent boredom as well as to receive value from each exercise for different parts of the body. All, however, benefit the cardiorespiratory system which is the basic need. I tore a cartilage in my knee several years ago while participating in sports, and by alternating the jogging with other activities that are nontraumatic to the joints, I rest my knee and it has not bothered me since it healed.

For most persons, we recommend walking/jogging as the form of aerobic activity for a basic exercise program. I recommend it not because it will produce greater benefits, but because of the following practical reasons. It is convenient because it can be done year-round without joining any clubs or classes. You can do it at home or away from home while on business trips or vacations. Your spouse, children, or neighbors may join you. Since no equipment other than good shoes is required, the cost is low. You can easily and quickly monitor your heart rate and adjust the rate of walking or jogging accordingly.

Practical Guidelines for a Walking/Jogging Program

1. *Shoes*. Shoes are of critical importance in jogging. Cost should not be a deterrent to buying good shoes. You can skimp on shorts and sweat suits but don't skimp on shoes. Of the 206 bones in the body, 52 are in the feet and ankles. The right shoes can prevent blisters, shin splints, and ankle, knee, and hip-joint problems.

They should have thick, wide soles and heels and a good cushion to absorb the shock of jogging. They should have a stable heel to prevent lateral movement of the foot (*pronation* and *supination*). The sole of the shoe should bend easily. The toes should have ample room to prevent toe problems and blisters. You should not jog in court shoes but in shoes made especially for jogging.

2. *Clothing*. Although clothing doesn't make the jogger, a jogger should give some consideration to clothing. The best overall jogging attire is shorts and a T-shirt. Warm-ups are often too warm to jog in. Women should wear a good bra with excellent support to prevent excessive bouncing of the breasts. A jogger should not wear rubberized or plastic clothing. Some persons wear this type of clothing to help in weight loss. However, the only weight lost as a result of wearing rubberized or plastic clothing is water loss, which may result in dehydration. Also, wearing such clothing prevents evaporation, therefore elevating body temperature, which can be harmful.

3. *Temperature and humidity.* Any time the temperature is above ninety degrees or above eighty degrees with humidity of 60 percent or more, you should slow your pace and consider jogging early in the morning or late in the evening. Also, before and after jogging in hot weather, you should drink a lot of water to compensate for water loss from excessive sweating. It is also desirable to drink during a long run in the heat.

In cold temperatures, you should wear gloves, a hat or hooded sweat shirt, sweat pants, and several tops that can be peeled off as you warm up. Long underwear is also excellent when jogging in cold weather. When the weather is very cold, that is, ten degrees or colder, you should wear a surgical or dental mask to warm the air before inhaling it. You need not fear the cold air on your lungs if you have no heart or lung disease. In a marathon in St. Paul, Minnesota, during February, more than two hundred runners ran the twenty-six miles in a temperature of minus ten degrees without a single respiratory problem reported. On the other hand, if you do have high blood pressure, heart disease, or asthma, you should avoid jogging in cold weather.

4. *Jogging surface.* You should jog on a surface that is smooth, has no holes or uneven spots, and has some spring in it. The best jogging surfaces, ranked from most to least desirable, are smooth and level grassy areas such as vacant lots or parks, running tracks, dirt roads, and asphalt. You should avoid jogging on cement since it is a hard surface and produces more wear and tear on the joints. Problems with running on grassy surfaces are unevenness and holes.

5. *Where and when to jog.* The safest places to jog are (1) running tracks, (2) large playgrounds, vacant lots, or parks, and (3) quiet side roads that are either dirt or asphalt. Remember, always jog facing traffic. Try to avoid jogging in heavy traffic since you inhale toxic fumes, increase your risk of being hit by a car, and annoy motorists.

Recently, while jogging on a street a well-known basketball coach was struck by a car and seriously injured. It occurred when he sidestepped a puddle in the street and stepped right into the path of a car. He violated two fundamental laws in jogging. First, he was jogging with the traffic rather than against it so he did not see the car. Second, he was wearing headphones and listening to a tape and didn't hear the car.

If you jog in hilly terrain, remember that it is always more difficult and demanding. The energy spent jogging up the hill is more than the energy saved when going down the hill. But don't try to speed up going down the hill, since the added jarring contributes to joint problems, especially in the low back, hips, and knees.

You should jog any time that is convenient and should program it into your schedule. The only consideration is that you should wait at least two hours after a moderate or heavy meal and one to one-and-a-half hours after a light meal. Joggers who tend to be most faithful jog early in the morning. Many others have found the noon hours to be a satisfactory time to jog. Others find a late-afternoon jog will give physiological as well as psychological benefits because of its value in relieving the tension and mental fatigue of the day. This is my favorite time to jog. However, the problem with jogging late in the afternoon is that it is too often possible for that time to be eroded by commitments of the day.

6. *Altitude.* In higher elevations the pressure of oxygen in the air decreases; therefore, less oxygen will be available to diffuse from your lungs into your blood stream and be delivered to your tissues. Above five thousand feet you need to slow your pace somewhat. If you live in the area for four to six weeks, your body will acclimatize to it and you can run at the same intensity and duration at that elevation as you did at sea level. The primary adjustment the body makes to allow this to take place is increasing the amount of hemoglobin and red blood cells in the blood to carry oxygen.

7. *Jogging form.* Jogging form is very important. You should stand up straight, lean forward slightly, and keep your head up. Resist the tendency to look at your feet or look just in front of your feet. Rather, look at least fifteen to twenty feet ahead of you. Although you should jog with good posture, don't be too rigid or your back muscles will become sore.

When jogging, you should land heel first, then roll to the ball of your foot, and push off from that point. Landing on the heel first cushions the blow of the landing, and rolling to the ball of the foot causes the jar to be distributed over the entire foot. This form of jogging will cause less wear and tear on your muscles and joints than landing flatfootedly or on the balls of your feet. Your arms should be bent slightly at the elbows and swing controllably backward and forward but should not cross the midline of your body.

While jogging, you should breathe normally and inhale and exhale slowly and deeply. By all means, breathe through your mouth, since at an overload of 65 percent to 85 percent of your maximum heart rate, you will not be able to get all the oxygen you need for your cells if you're breathing only through your nose.

8. *Overfat.* A considerably obese person (a woman over 30 percent or a man over 20 percent fat) will have a greater tendency toward joint problems and muscle soreness from a jogging program because of the excess jarring on the joints. For this reason, an overfat person should progress more gradually into jogging. The first objective should be to lose weight through a good diet, and the first forms of exercise should be walking,

cycling, or swimming, not jogging. We will discuss this more in chapter 15.

9. *Warm-up, activity, cool-down.* Any activity program should consist of three basic parts: warm-up, the actual activity, and cool-down. The warm-up should consist of five to ten minutes of stretching exercises, calisthenics, and walking. During this time all the joints and muscles of the body are moved so as to increase the muscle and body temperature several degrees. This will increase skeletal muscular contraction and increase the circulation of blood to the muscles. You will perform the activity more efficiently and will be less likely to pull a muscle or tendon.

Warm-up also increases the fluid to the articulating cartilage of the joint and therefore provides a better cushion during the exercise. This makes the joint less susceptible to trauma, resulting in fewer joint injuries. Also, fewer ECG abnormalities occur during exercise following a warm-up.

The second part of the exercise routine consists of the actual activity, whether cycling, jogging, swimming, or whatever. This is when the actual overload is placed upon the system and the primary cardiorespiratory benefits occur.

The third part of the activity routine is the cool-down. This is important because research has found that if a person is jogging or cycling, as much as 80 percent of the blood volume is transmitted or directed to the legs. Therefore if a person stops abruptly, much of that blood will remain in or pool in the legs. This will reduce the amount of blood flowing back to the heart, which will reduce the amount of blood flow to the brain and may cause dizziness or fainting. A cool-down of walking, light cycling, or slowing down whatever you were doing is beneficial in returning your body to a normal state after the activity. The cool-down period should last for three to five minutes, depending upon the intensity of the exercise. The more intense the exercise, the longer the cool-down should be.

10. *Rest.* The tissues of the body respond to exercise in an interesting and unusual way. In response to the exercise stimulus, if the overload is sufficient, there will be some breakdown of the exercised muscles. Then, as you rest, the muscles overcompensate for what was broken down during the exercise, and they build stronger cells and tissues. However, time must be allowed for the muscles to rejuvenate. Therefore, to prevent injuries and to allow the muscles to rejuvenate and become stronger you should allow at least twenty-four hours between normal exercise workouts and forty-eight hours between hard workouts.

We recognize that many topflight endurance athletes exercise every day and occasionally twice a day. Rarely, however, will the workouts be hard two days in a row. It is also important to remember that these persons have taken years to develop their bodies to handle this type of stress. The average person, especially one who is just developing health fitness, could prevent many potential injuries by allowing time between workouts as indicated here.

While some persons exercise too often and too intensely without sufficient rest between exercise bouts, others exercise too seldom and are prone to injuries. If you participate in physical activities on the weekends only, you may do more harm than good to your body.

A Test of Cardiorespiratory Fitness

We have said a goal of your fitness program should be to exercise aerobically three to six days per week at 85 percent for thirty minutes, 75 percent for forty-five minutes, or 65 percent for sixty minutes. When you have achieved this goal in your walking/jogging program, but *not before*, you may want to test your cardiorespiratory fitness by a performance test. (As previously mentioned, do not attempt a performance test unless cleared by your physician.)

An excellent test of your cardiorespiratory fitness is a three-mile walk/jog, a six-mile outdoor cycle, or an eleven-hundred-meter swim. You can classify the health fitness of your cardiorespiratory system on the basis of this test. The jogging and cycling should be done on a flat track. The cycling can be done with a five- to ten-speed bike. The standard for swimming is based upon a swimmer with above average skill.

TABLE 9.1
Level of Cardiorespiratory Fitness According to Time on 3-mile Jog, 6-mile Cycle, or 1100-meter Swim in Minutes

LEVEL OF CARDIO-RESPIRATORY FITNESS	MEN				WOMEN			
	AGE				AGE			
	25	25–40	40–55	55–70	25	25–40	40–55	55–70
Superior	18:00	19:00	21:00	24:00	21:00	22:00	24:00	27:00
Excellent	21:00	22:00	24:00	26:00	24:00	25:00	27:00	29:00
Good	23:00	24:00	26:00	29:00	26:00	27:00	29:00	32:00
Fair	25:00	27:00	29:00	33:00	28:00	30:00	32:00	36:00
Poor	27:00	30:00	33:00	36:00	30:00	33:00	36:00	39:00
Very Poor	27:00+	30:00+	33:00+	36:00+	30:00+	33:00+	36:00+	39:00+

Steps You Could Take

1. What will be the best aerobic exercise for you to do, considering your needs and interests and the availability of the activity?

2. What precautions will you follow to have a successful exercise program?

3. In chapter 8, application 5, you listed your heart rate and duration goals. Now list what activities you will do and the number of days each week you will do them. Remember you should exercise three to six days per week every week.

10

Exercises for the Muscular-skeletal System

We have been emphasizing aerobic exercises for the development of the cardiorespiratory system. That is because the fitness of this system is paramount in order to have optimal health and well-being and to prevent heart disease. However, we don't want to ignore the need for fitness of the skeletal muscles of the body. When we ignore those muscles, the results can be muscle weakness, back pain, and excess body fat. The skeletal muscles are attached to the bones. We control them voluntarily, and when they contract, they cause movement of the body.

The body has more than four hundred skeletal muscles, which account for about 45 percent of the male's body weight and 35 percent of the female's. This can vary according to a person's health fitness, as is discussed in chapter 13. Each muscle is made up of thousands of individual muscle fibers, each surrounded by connective tissue. The connective tissue comes together at the end of the muscle to form a tendon, which is attached to a bone.

When the brain wants a certain movement, a nerve impulse is sent to the appropriate muscles. When the impulse arrives, the muscles act as a machine, converting chemical energy into mechanical energy. The muscle fibers contract (shorten) and cause a pull on the connective tissue which in turn pulls the tendon which pulls the bone. If the force generated by the muscle is greater than the resistance offered by the bone, the bone moves.

The need for our muscles to be fit is somewhat obvious. It is basic to satisfactory performance in all sports and athletic activities. It is basic to such routine daily tasks as carrying an armful of books across campus, climbing a flight of stairs with a suitcase or a sack of groceries, moving furniture around the room, carrying a baby from store to store while shopping, preventing fatigue in the fingers when taking notes or typing, pushing a stalled car, or changing a tire. In addition to these needs for fitness in the muscular-skeletal system, perhaps the greatest need is for the prevention of injury and low-back problems.

Muscle-development Exercises

Basically two types of exercises develop and maintain fitness of the muscles: (1) stretching exercises are essential for muscle and tendon *flexibility*, and (2) strengthening exercises are essential for muscle *strength* and tone. Stretching exercises will not produce strength, and strengthening exercises will not produce flexibility. Therefore, both must be done.

Flexibility

Flexibility is the ability of the muscle and tendon to allow a joint to move through its entire range of motion. Muscles that lack flexibility prohibit complete joint movement and make individuals susceptible to muscle tears and back pain.

Although you could test the flexibility of all your joints, a simple test that is indicative of your body's flexibility is the *sit-and-reach test*. To take this test, sit on the floor with your knees fully extended. Reach forward as far as possible with both hands, keeping your legs and the back of your knees flat against the floor. Hold for three seconds and *don't bounce!* The following table reflects the flexibility of your low-back and hamstring muscles (back of the legs) on the basis of this test.

TABLE 10.1
Sit-and-reach Flexibility Test

FLEXIBILITY CATEGORY	INCHES REACHED
Excellent	More than 4 inches beyond the toes
Good	Touching toes to 4 inches beyond toes
Fair	Within 2 inches of touching toes
Poor	Within 3 to 5 inches of touching toes
Very Poor	More than 5 inches from the toes

Stretching for Flexibility

A variety of different stretching exercises can improve your flexibility. I recommend that you do the following ones which are for the calf, thighs, hips, low back, shoulders, and neck. They should be performed daily, if possible, but at *least three days per week*. Include them in your warm-up and repeat them again in your cool-down. Or do them while watching TV or listening to tapes. Do each exercise slowly and precisely. *Never bounce*. Stretch gradually to the point of discomfort and then hold for ten to thirty seconds. Repeat three to five times.

Fig. 10.1. Neck Stretch

1. *Neck*. Stand with your feet wider apart than your shoulders, your hands on your hips, or sit upright in a straight-back chair. Roll your chin on your chest and around in as wide a circle as possible. Complete three circles slowly in each direction.

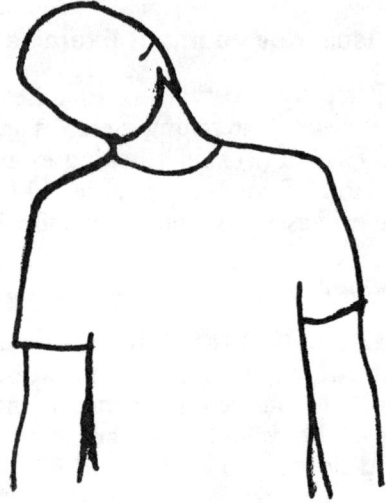

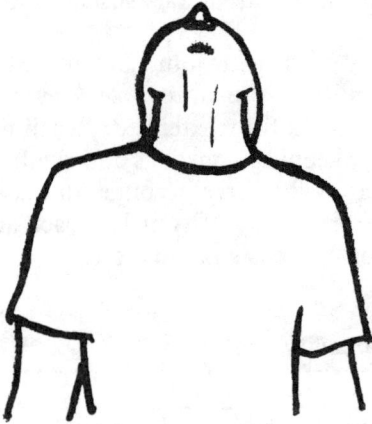

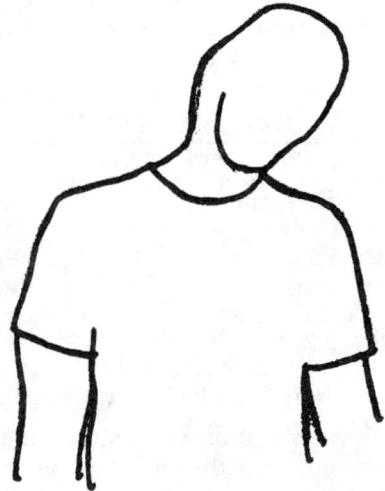

Fig. 10.2. Shoulder Stretch 1

2. *Shoulder*
   a. Stand with your feet shoulder width apart, your arms at your sides. Put your arms behind you and interlace your fingers. Now, rotate your palms down, straighten your elbows, and raise your arms.

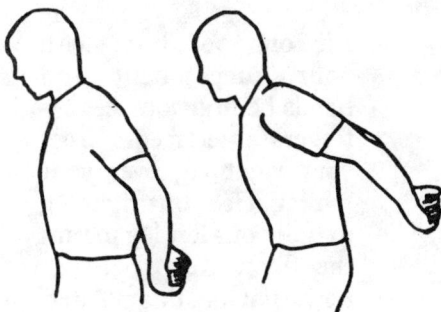

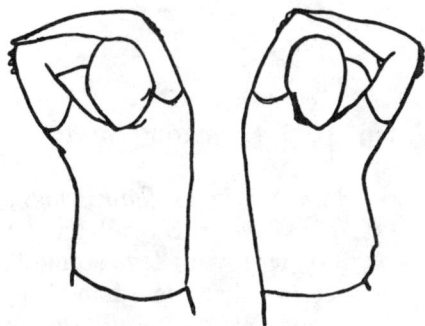

Fig. 10.3. Shoulder Stretch 2

   b. Stand with your feet shoulder width apart and fold your arms behind your head. With one hand on opposite elbow, pull arm gently. Alternate sides.

Fig. 10.4. Low-back Stretch 1

3. *Low back and hips*
   a. Lie on your back with your legs straight. Raise your right knee and pull it with your hands to your chest as far as you can. Repeat with left knee, and then do both knees together.

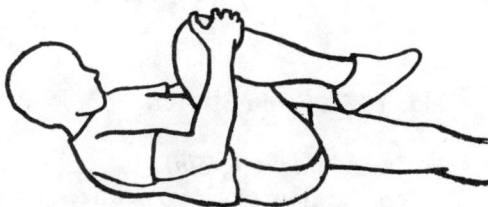

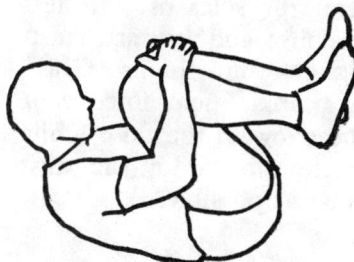

Fig. 10.5. Low-back Stretch 2

b. Lie on your back with your knees bent and hands behind your head—fingers interlaced. Cross your right leg over your left leg. Use your right leg to pull your left leg toward the floor. Keep both elbows flat on floor. Alternate legs.

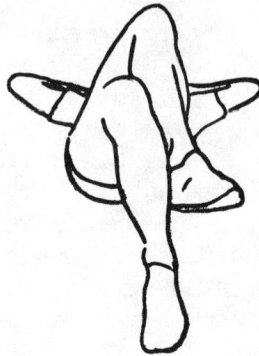

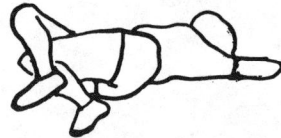

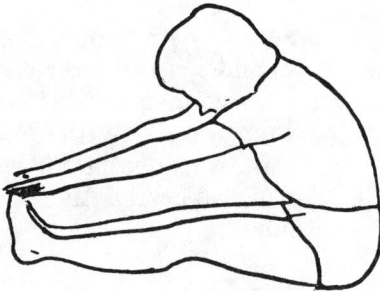

Fig. 10.6. Hamstring Stretch

4. *Back of thighs (hamstrings), sit and reach.* Sit tall on the floor with your legs straight, feet together, and hands on thighs. Bend forward slowly at the waist and reach your fingers toward your toes.

Fig. 10.7. Groin Stretch

5. *Inside thighs (groin).* Sit tall on the floor with your knees bent, the soles of your feet touching, and your arms resting on your thighs. Grasp your ankles and force your knees toward the floor while bending forward at the waist as far as possible.

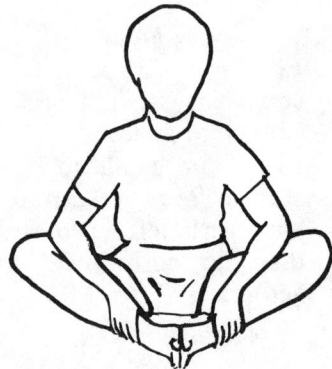

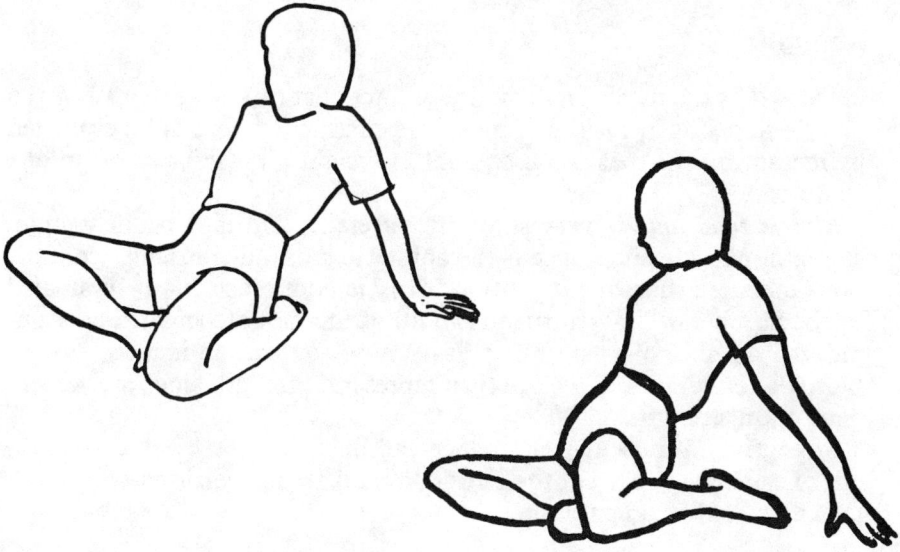

Fig. 10.8. Quadriceps Stretch

6. *Upper thighs (quadriceps)*. Sit on the floor with your right leg bent. Your left leg is also bent, and the side of your left foot is on your right knee. Slowly lean backward, alternate side.

   Lie backward and attempt to lie flat while keeping your knee flat on the floor. Hold for five seconds. Avoid bouncing movements. Switch legs and repeat five times on each side.

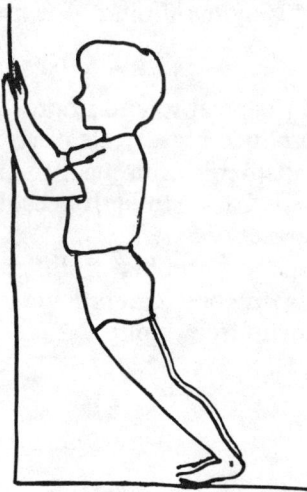

Fig. 10.9. Calf Stretch

7. *Calf*. Stand straight and erect with your palms against a wall at about eye level. Step backward one to one-and-a-half yards from the wall, supporting your weight on your hands. Stay flatfooted until you feel your calf muscles stretch.

Strength

Strength is the maximum amount of force that can be generated by the muscle in a single, maximal, muscular contraction. It can be evaluated by measuring the maximum amount of weight a person can lift in one contraction.

Muscle endurance is very similar to strength and is dependent upon strength. Muscle endurance is the ability to continue muscular contractions for more than one repetition. Muscle endurance can be evaluated by the number of times a person can lift an amount of weight. For example, the number of pushups or situps a person can do is a measure of muscular endurance, which in turn represents strength since it is dependent upon strength.

Strength and muscular endurance can be developed by several methods of exercises. Three of the most common are isometric exercises, calisthenics, and weight training.

Isometric Exercises

An isometric exercise is one in which the muscles contract at near maximum force, but no movement of the limb or body occurs. This is because the muscles contract while you attempt to lift or move some immovable object, such as a wall, doorway, heavy chair, heavy weights, another person, or parts of your own body. Although isometric exercises have some value, they will not result in as much benefit as the next two exercise methods. They also have a negative side effect in that the blood pressure is elevated during the exercise. Therefore, do isometric exercises only when you can't do either weight training or calisthenics.

Calisthenics

Calisthenics are a convenient and practical way to improve and maintain your strength. They will not produce high levels of strength (only weight training will do that), but calisthenics can meet the need of the average person who desires to have the basic strength necessary to have good health and fitness in the skeletal muscles.

As was true for stretching exercises, the number of different kinds of calisthenics is tremendous. The following ones can provide you with the basic strength you need in the major muscle groups.

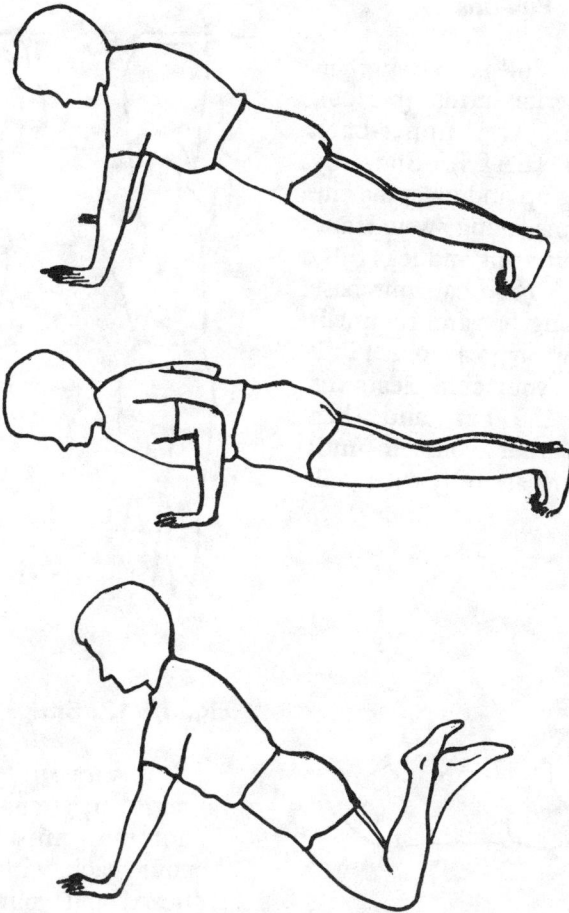

Fig. 10.10. Pushups

1. *Pushups.* Pushups can strengthen the posterior arms (triceps), chest (pectoralis), and shoulder muscle (deltoid). Start with your body straight and your hands shoulder width apart, fingers pointing forward. Straighten your elbows and support your weight on your hands and toes. (Persons who can't do a regular pushup can support their weight on their hands and knees if necessary.) Then lower your body by bending your elbows and touching your chest to the floor while keeping your head up and your back straight. Be sure your elbows are extended with each repetition.

Fig. 10.11. Pull-ups

2. *Pull-ups.* Pull-ups strengthen the anterior arms (biceps), shoulder, and upper-back muscles (LATS). Start by jumping up and grasping the bar, palms facing away. Hang with your arms and legs fully extended. (You can purchase a chinning bar and mount it in a doorway to a closet.) Pull up until your chin clears the top of the bar, and then slowly lower yourself until your arms are fully extended.

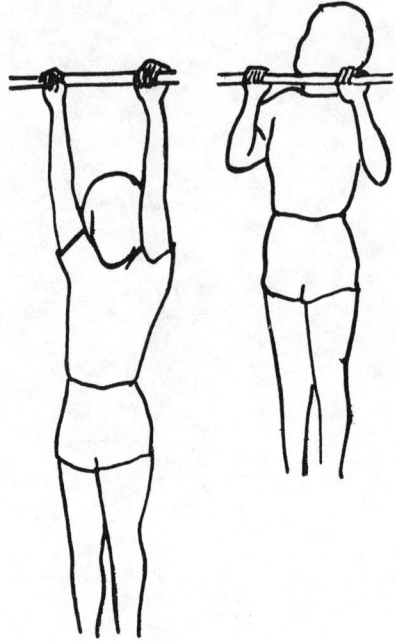

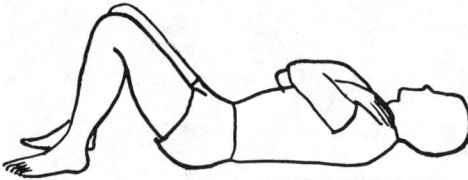

Fig. 10.12. Situps

3. *Bent knee situps.* The situp serves to strengthen the abdominal muscles. Lie on your back with your knees flexed and your feet flat on the floor. Your feet should be held by a partner or hooked under a chair. Cross your hands across your chest and hold your shoulders. Sit up by lifting your head and shoulders, and roll up until your elbows touch your knees. Avoid this exercise if you have back trouble (see chap. 11).

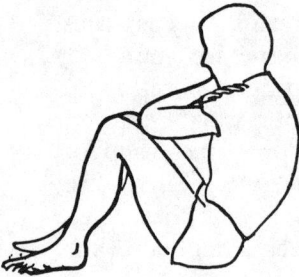

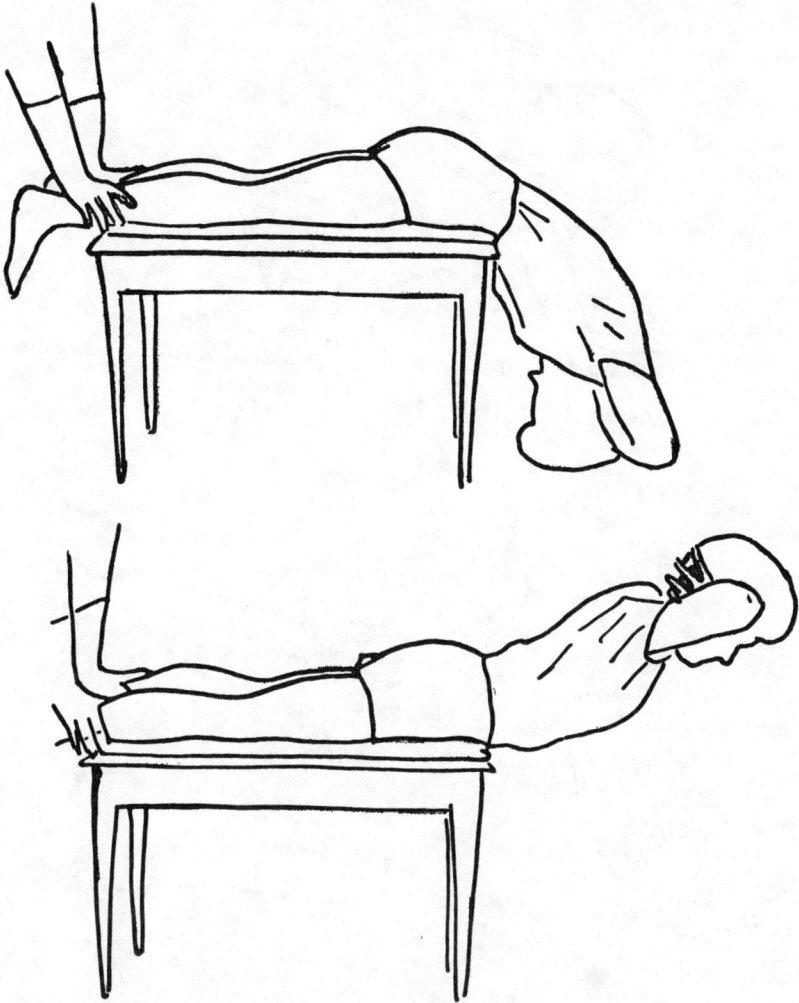

Fig. 10.13. Back Extensions

4. *Back extensions.* Back extensions are to strengthen back muscles
   supporting the vertebral column. Lie on your stomach on a table or
   a bed, letting your upper body lean over while a partner holds your
   feet down. Place your hands behind your head. Lower your upper
   body toward the floor and then raise it up again. Avoid this exercise
   if you have back trouble (see chap. 11).

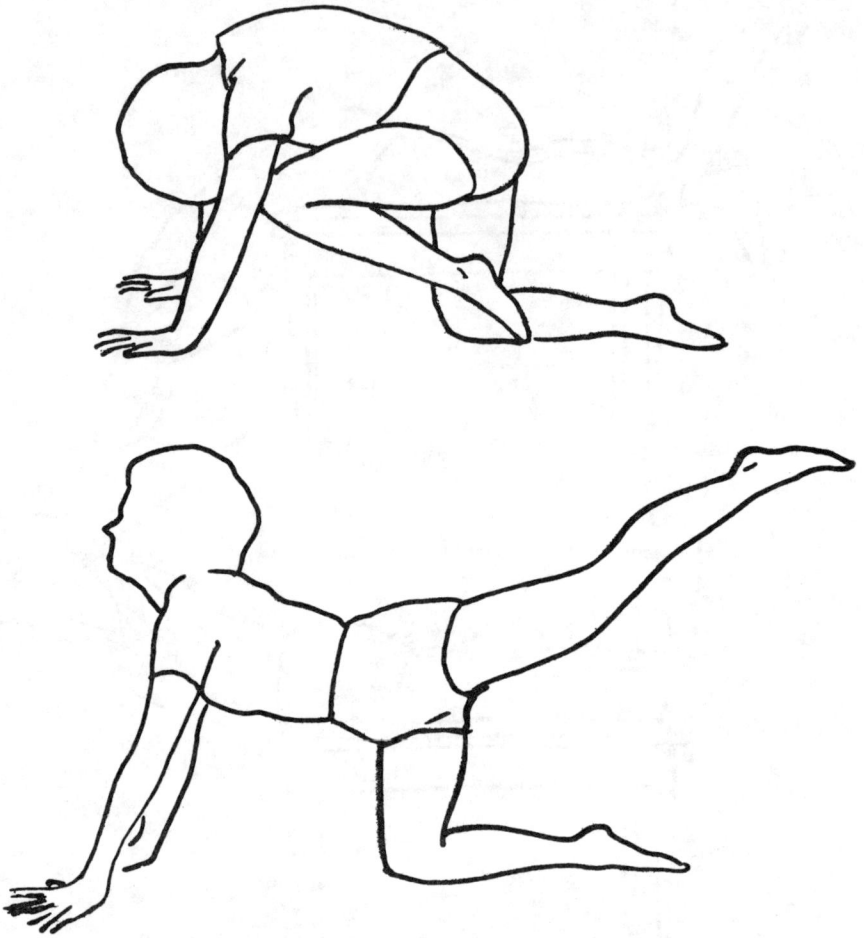

Fig. 10.14. Donkey Kicks

5. *Donkey kicks.* This exercise functions to strengthen the low back and buttocks. From a hands-and-knees position on the floor, lower your head and bring your right knee to your forehead. Then, slowly raise your head while stretching your right leg backward and straightening your knee. Then raise both your head and your leg as high as possible. Return to the starting position, and repeat with your right leg as many times as desired. Then repeat with your left leg.

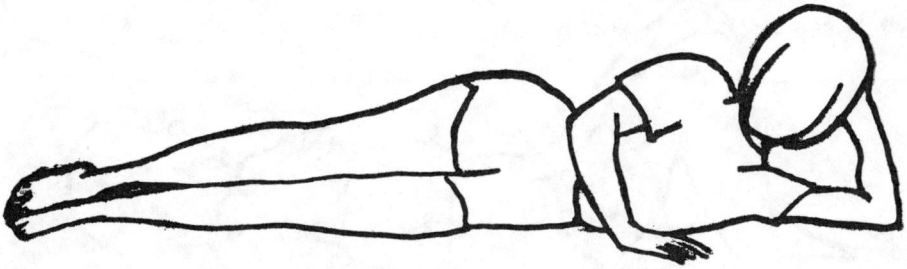

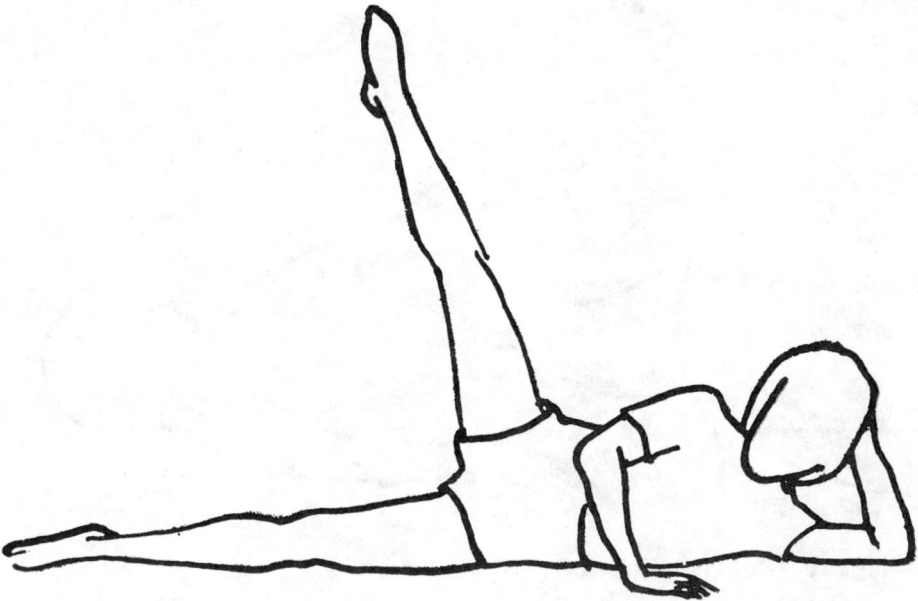

Fig. 10.15. Side Leg Raises

6. *Side leg raises*. These function to strengthen lateral thigh, posterior hip muscles, and muscles on the sides that support the vertebral column. Lie on your side with your head resting on your hand. Raise your leg laterally as high as possible, keeping your knee straight and your hip pushed forward. Move your leg slowly up and down.

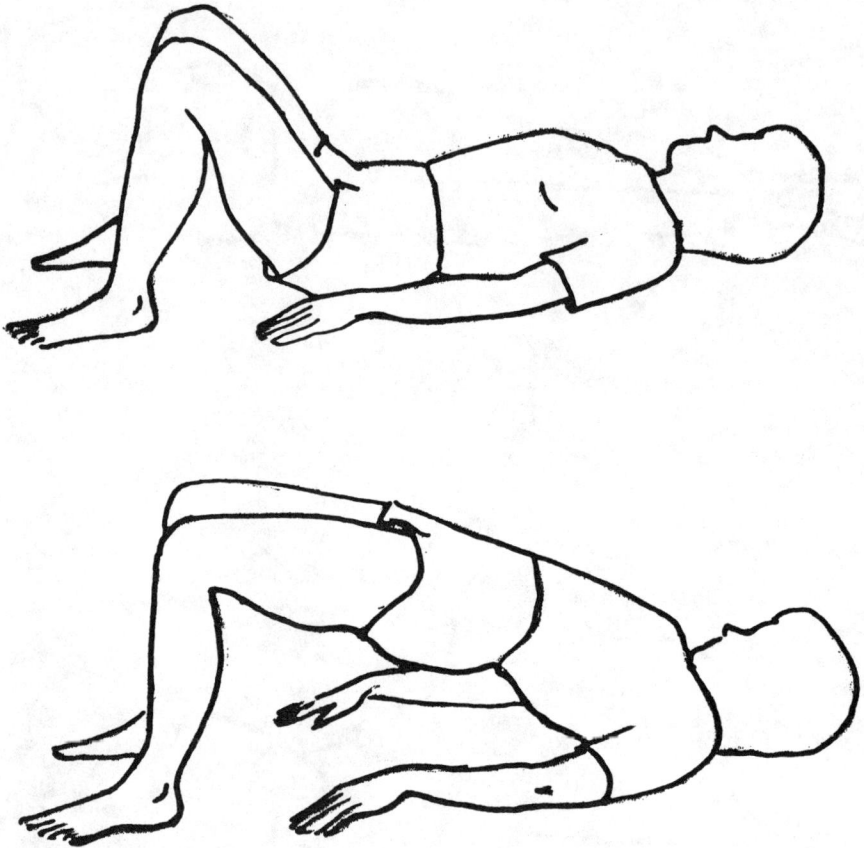

Fig. 10.16. Pelvic Raises

7. *Pelvic raises.* Pelvic raises strengthen the gluteal muscles of the buttock, which will provide stability to the low back. Lie on your back with your knees flexed and feet flat on the floor, your hands at your sides on the floor. Raise your pelvis up as high as possible by contracting the gluteal muscles and then lower pelvis to the floor.

Repetition goal for calisthenics. As in the case of a walking/jogging program, you should begin easily, exercising three times per week and gradually increasing the number of repetitions. The following table represents a goal to strive for on the basis of strength and muscular endurance you desire. All exercises are repeated without stopping to increase your level of fitness.

TABLE 10.2
Calisthenics Repetitions and Fitness

LEVEL OF MUSCULAR FITNESS	PUSH-UPS[a]	PULL-UPS[b]		SIT-UPS	BACK EXTENSIONS	DONKEY KICKS (EACH LEG)	SIDE LEG RAISES	PELVIC RAISES
Excellent	50	12	6	60	20	40	60	60
Good	30	9	3	45	14	30	50	50
Fair	20	6	2	25	8	20	30	30
Poor	15	4	1	20	4	10	20	20
Very Poor fewer than	15	4	1	20	4	10	20	20

[a] Standards for men and women are the same, but women can do modified style pushups.

[b] The second column represents pull-ups for women.

Lead-up calisthenics. If you can't do a single situp or pushup, don't feel bad. I often find in the seminars I present and in the freshmen who come to ORU that some persons have let their fitness deteriorate to the extent that they cannot perform a single situp or pushup, let alone try to do a pull-up. Don't give up. Modify the regular calisthenics to do what you can.

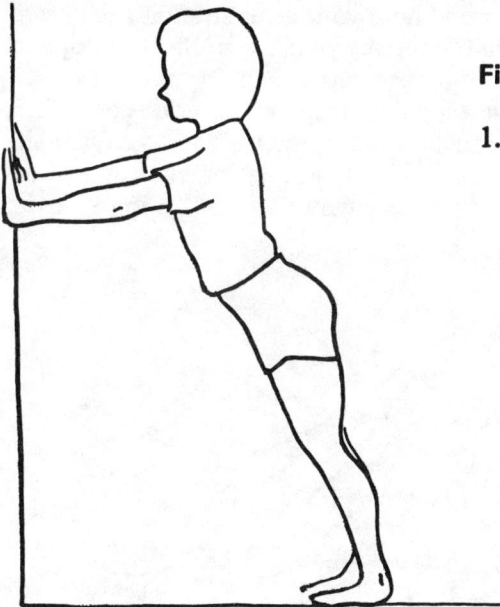

Fig. 10.17. Lead-up Pushup

1. *Lead-up pushup.* Stand a little beyond your arm's reach from a wall. Then reach out and place your hands about shoulder height on the wall. Lean forward until your chest almost touches the wall and then push away and return to the starting position.

When you build up to being able to do forty of these, then lower your hands on the wall and stand back farther from the wall. When you can do forty at this level, perform

the pushups on the back of a
chair, then the seat of a chair,
and finally you'll be able to
do them on the floor on your
knees first and later on your
toes.

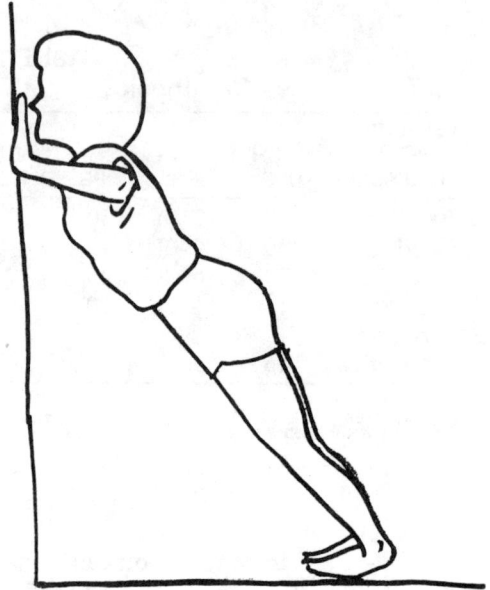

Fig. 10.18. Lead-up Situp

2. *Curl-up situp.* Lie on your back on the floor with your knees bent.
Hook your thumbs together and hold your arms straight out toward
your knees. Raise your head, contract your stomach muscles, and
reach up until you touch your knee caps, then let yourself down.
Gradually do more of these each day until you can do sixty. Then
you probably will have enough abdominal strength to do regular situps. We call this exercise "curl-ups." It is an extremely valuable exercise for persons with back trouble, which we will discuss in the
next chapter.

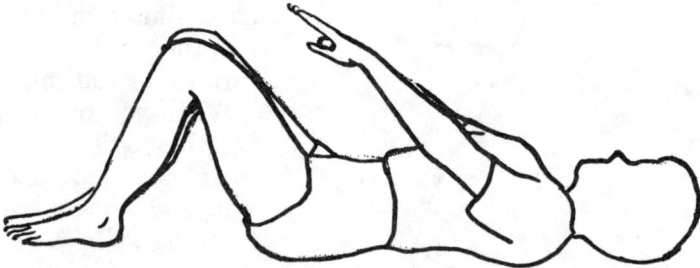

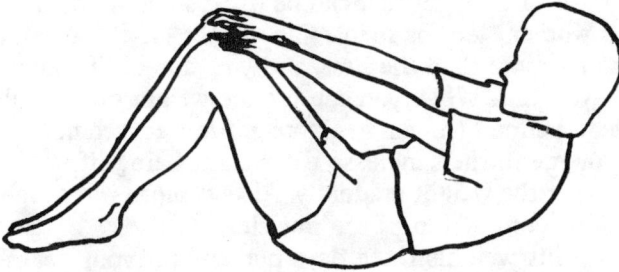

Weight Training

Weight training is the best exercise method to increase the strength of your muscles. You can control the weight being lifted so that you receive maximum benefit, and you can perform numerous exercises for nearly every muscle in your body. The only drawback to weight training is that you need a set of weights at home or you must have access to weights at a fitness center.

The following guidelines are given for persons (*both* men and women) who choose to exercise their muscles by weight training. Women need not fear developing bulky muscles. The program is aimed at a combination of developing both strength and muscular endurance.

1. Warm up before weight training (stretch and walk).

2. First perform all the exercises in Circuit 1 in the order listed, then do Circuit 2.

TABLE 10.3
Guidelines for Weight Training

EXERCISES	CIRCUIT 1 REPETITIONS		CIRCUIT 2 REPETITIONS
	WOMEN	MEN	
Bench press	15	10	As many as possible
Lat pull	15	10	As many as possible
*Situps			
*Pelvic raises			
Elbow extensions	15	10	As many as possible
Arm curls	15	10	As many as possible
Knee curls	15	10	As many as possible
Knee extensions	15	10	As many as possible

*Situps and pelvic raises were discussed under calisthenics section.

3. The weight lifted for the first circuit at each exercise should be selected on the basis of a weight that can be lifted some with difficulty fifteen times for women, ten for men. The weight for the second circuit should be slightly more than the first, and you should lift the weight as many times as you can. When you can lift the weight on a regular basis during the second circuit (fifteen to eighteen times for women and ten to twelve times for men), then increase the weight being lifted.

4. Lift and lower the weight gradually. Always move it through a complete range of the contraction of the muscle.

5. You should lift weights three days per week if your goal is to improve. Always allow forty-eight hours between weightlifting workouts. This allows your muscles the opportunity to recover from the previous workout. Once you develop an adequate amount of strength, weight training once per week will maintain it.

6. If you desire to enter into a full-fledged body-building program, the basic program given here would need to be expanded. Consult with trained personnel in this area for assistance.

Muscle Hypertrophy (Enlargement)

People want to know if their muscles will get larger if they do muscle exercises (weight training or calisthenics). Many men have this desire, and most women don't. The answer is dependent upon several variables.

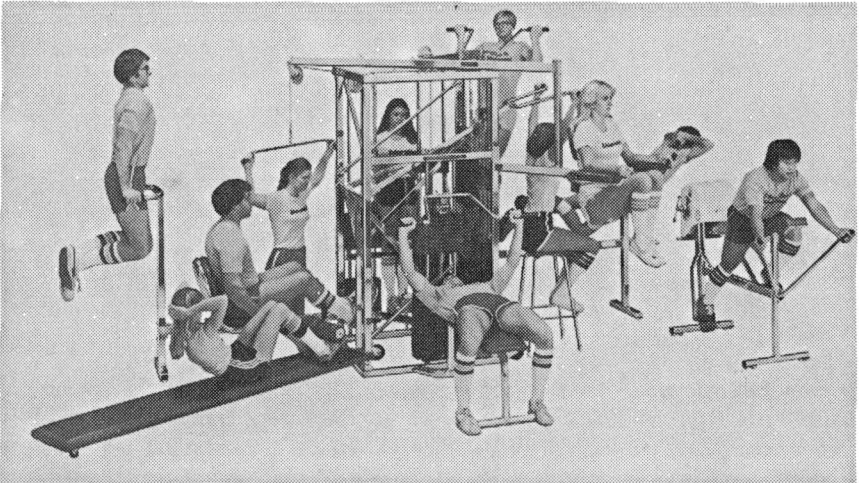

Fitness centers can offer a variety of equipment for weight training not normally available for home use.

Photo courtesy of Universal Gym Equipment, Inc., Cedar Rapids, Iowa.

In an average person, 50 percent or less of the muscle fibers are functional and 50 percent or more are latent, or nonfunctional. One of the first effects of a muscle-training program is an increase in the number of functional fibers in the muscle. Therefore, a well-conditioned person may have 75 percent to 90 percent of muscle fibers functional with only 10 percent to 25 percent latent. This added number of muscle fibers responding to a nervous impulse to contract greatly increases the strength of the muscle without any increase in muscle size.

Once approximately 90 percent of the muscle fibers are functional, then the stimulus of the muscle-training program will cause the functional muscle fibers to begin to grow larger. Therefore, at the onset of a conditioning program considerable strength may be gained in the first six to twelve weeks before there is any muscle hypertrophy. This is because it takes at least this long for latent fibers to become functional.

A male who wants to increase the bulk of his muscles and starts a conditioning program should not expect a large increase in bulk for at least twelve weeks because it may take that long for him to have 75 percent to 95 percent of his muscle fibers functional. Only then will the functional fibers begin to increase in size and only if he begins to use heavier weights and few repetitions (six to ten repetitions rather than ten to fifteen and three or four sets rather than two).

With regard to a woman's fear of getting large, bulky muscles, research has shown that a woman can increase strength as much as 75 percent to 100 percent without any increase in muscle size. This is because women are protected by the hormone estrogen and lack the male hormone testosterone. Testosterone stimulates muscle growth and causes the muscles to increase in size. Therefore, a man and a woman using two identical conditioning programs will both increase in strength, but after both muscles are using 90 percent of the muscle fibers, the man's muscle size will increase and the woman's will not. Donna can do forty men's pushups but is slim and trim muscularly.

Steps You Could Take

1. Perform stretching exercises at least three days per week. Remember to perform them slowly, never bounce.

2. If weights are available, set up a weight-training program and experiment to determine the appropriate weight for Circuit 1 and Circuit 2.

3 .Take the strength and muscle endurance tests. Score the number you did and record the level of muscular fitness.

	WEIGHT FOR CIRCUIT 1	WEIGHT FOR CIRCUIT 2
Bench Press	_____	_____
Lat Pull	_____	_____
Elbow Extensions	_____	_____
Arm Curls	_____	_____
Knee Curls	_____	_____
Knee Extensions	_____	_____

	NUMBER	MUSCULAR FITNESS LEVEL
Pushups	_____	_____
Pull-ups	_____	_____
Situps	_____	_____
*Back Extensions	_____	_____
Donkey Kicks	R L _____	_____
Side Leg Raises	R L _____	_____
Pelvic Raises	_____	_____

*Do not take the test to maximum if you have any back trouble.

4 .If you have weights available and are following a weight-training program, add situps and pelvic raises to the circuit. Do at least three days per week.

	NUMBER TO PERFORM THE FIRST WEEK	NUMBER TO ADD EACH WEEK
Situps	_____	_____
Pelvic Raises	_____	_____

5 .If weights are not available, set up a calisthenic program. Do as many as you can of each calisthenic listed, three days per week, until you achieve the level of muscular fitness you desire. Then do the exercises once a week to maintain that level.

11

No More Backaches

Most adults seem to experience some form of low-back pain during their lifetimes. Of the adult population 80 percent are estimated to have suffered from low-back problems at one time or another. Back problems account for more lost man-hours than any other occupational injury and consequently account for a significant portion of the mounting health costs. In the search for a healthy back Americans spend more than $5 billion a year for tests and treatments from orthopedic physicians, osteopaths, physical therapists, and chiropractors.

Oh, My Aching Back!

Back problems can take several forms. The pain may result from pathological problems such as arthritis, rheumatism, a cancerous tumor growing on the spine, osteoporosis, or infection. It may result from a fall, a blow to the spinal column, or pregnancy. But the vast majority (80 percent) of back problems are not caused by any of these reasons. Instead, they are due to muscle deficiency caused by an inappropriate lifestyle. Three of the most common back problems are back strains, back sprains, and the infamous "slipped disc."

Back Strain

The most common back problem is the back strain, which usually is the result of working hard in the garden, moving the furniture, or undertaking some other physical activity in which the back muscles were asked to do more than they were capable of doing at that moment. The strained muscles or tendons cause inflammation, fluids build-up, muscle spasms, and painful pressure on the nerve endings. The muscle spasms constrict the blood vessels and further complicate the problem by not allowing blood, oxygen, and nutrients to reach the area or waste products to be carried off.

The immediate treatment for a back strain is rest, aspirin to reduce the inflammation, and perhaps a muscle relaxant prescribed by a physician to relax the muscle spasm. Usually in a few days the pain will be gone—*but*—it will return if you don't begin a preventive program.

Back Sprain

A back sprain is very similar to a back strain but is more severe. Whereas a strain usually doesn't involve a muscle tear, a sprain occurs when a muscle, a tendon, or a ligament has actually torn. All the same factors occur as in a strain, but the pain is more acute and the recovery will take longer. Often the sprain results when a weakened or inflexible muscle is called upon rather suddenly to do something it is not capable of doing. Lifting a heavy object, swinging a golf club the wrong way, or moving in some slight way could cause a muscle sprain. Perhaps you had a stressful day, tension mounted, your muscles were tight, you moved just the wrong way, and...*zap*!!

The immediate treatment for a sprain is the same as for a strain. The recovery will take longer, and the injured area will not be as good as new. A weakness in that area will be susceptible to a repeat performance, usually of greater severity, unless you begin a preventive program.

"Slipped Disc"

Although a slipped disc is the most-talked-about back ailment, it accounts for only 5 percent of back problems. Back strains and sprains account for the other 95 percent. If a back sprain is severe enough, it can mimic a slipped disc.

A slipped disc is technically not slipped. It has not slipped out so it cannot slip back in. The cartilage that serves as a cushion between the vertebrae is known as a disc. When excess pressure is placed upon the disc, it may *herniate* (rupture). When this occurs, some of the jellylike center of the disc bulges out of the disc and pushes against the nerves in the spinal cord. These nerves are extremely sensitive, and the least pressure against them triggers often excruciating pain.

A long history of repeated attacks of muscle strains and sprains can begin the process of disc deterioration. Initially the disc deterioration may cause no symptoms and may go unnoticed. This process may eventually lead to a ruptured disc. Although a ruptured disc is often difficult to diagnose, two symptoms are usually present. First, since the most common location of the problem is in the low back, the sciatic nerve usually has pressure placed upon it. This will cause pain (called *sciatica*) going down one or both of the legs. If there is no pain down the leg, the back problem is probably not a disc rupture.

The second symptom can be tested in the following manner. Lie flat on your back on the floor. Have someone lift one of your legs at a time. If the straight leg can be lifted up seventy to eighty degrees or more without any pain in your low back, this would be a sign of no ruptured disc. This test, however, should not be done when you have any significant degree of spasms in your back. If, on the other hand, your straight leg can be lifted only twenty or thirty degrees before you feel pain (the foot being perhaps two feet off the floor), this is an indication of a possible ruptured disc. If this pain is present, you should see your doctor.

Treatment for a ruptured disc—case history. Very often a ruptured disc requires surgery. However, unless you change your lifestyle the problem will return following your recovery from surgery. It is possible for a ruptured disc to heal in time without surgery and not recur if you make a significant lifestyle change.

A close personal friend and jogging and sports companion had suffered occasional bouts of pain for longer than ten years. He was in excellent aerobic condition and jogged fifteen to twenty miles a week. He was a superb athlete but was inconsistent in his back exercise program. After a bout of back pain that would lay him low for several days, he would return to his back exercises. He would then be faithful for several weeks. As his back strengthened and the pain disappeared, he would begin to ignore the back exercises. *Zap*—it would hit him again.

As time progressed, the back problems were becoming more severe and more frequent. Finally, the disc deteriorated to the point of rupture. He didn't believe it at first, but after three different physicians made the same diagnosis, he was convinced.

According to the diagnosis, the reason for the disc's rupturing in his case was fourfold:

1. He did not follow a regular back exercise program.
2. He engaged in numerous physical activities that had the potential of being hard on a weak back, sports with a lot of twisting and turning such as racquetball, tennis, and basketball.
3. He was having back pain more frequently, and he did not heed the warnings and correct his lifestyle.
4. Even though he was in overall excellent physical condition, the doctors discovered through X rays that he had been born with a form of spina bifida, a problem of which he was unaware. The spinous process of his top vertebra of the sacrum was missing. This meant that the small muscles which cross the sacroiliac joint had no place for attachment. Therefore, a weakness at that joint partially added

to the problem. (Approximately 10 percent of back problems are caused by a missing spinous process.)

Usually a person with the spina bifida problem will need a back brace and/or surgery before age thirty. Since our friend was in excellent overall condition, he had made it to age forty before the problem became severe. Because of his good fitness, the decision was to first treat his back nonsurgically. The treatment involved complete bed rest for two weeks and anti-inflammatants, followed by several months of limited activity.

Fortunately this treatment was successful. It took three months for the sciatica to completely heal and six months before the flexibility completely returned. But, what is more important, only a minor change in his lifestyle has kept the severe pain away for more than four years. Surgery can be prevented for many back pain sufferers.

Aspects of Exercise for the Back

Exercises for the low back must consist of both calisthenics for strength and stretching for flexibility.

Strength

Four specific muscle groups that support the vertebral column, the pelvis, and the abdomen must have good strength. The *back muscles* support the entire vertebral column and must be strong. If they are weak, when performing heavy work they will be strained and cause back pain.

The *abdominal muscles* must be strong to keep the pelvis tilted up and prevent it from rotating down (giving a potbelly or swayback appearance). When the pelvis is rotated down, undesirable pressure is placed on the vertebrae of the low back, the discs, and the nerves that branch from the spinal cord to the muscles in the low-back area and legs.

The *gluteal muscles* are also important for stabilizing the pelvis. They are attached to the back of the pelvis and the upper part of the back of the thigh. They also assist in preventing the pelvis from rotating down in front.

Finally, the *iliopsoas muscles* must be strong and flexible. This muscle group has as its upper attachment the inside of the vertebral column of the low back and runs through the pelvic girdle and is attached to the front of the upper thigh. You cannot see this muscle. It is a muscle group that is important in hip flexion and also supports and stabilizes the lower part of the back.

Flexibility

Key muscle groups in the body which keep us upright are always mildly contracting when we are sitting, standing, walking, or jogging.

Because they are mildly contracted for much of the day, they will develop tightness if we do not specifically stretch them out to increase flexibility.

The back muscles, the hamstring muscle group (located in back of the thighs and attached at the lower end below the knee and at the upper end to the back of the pelvis), and the iliopsoas muscle are three such muscle groups. For example, when we are sitting down, as we are so much of the time, the iliopsoas muscle is in a shortened state. Upon standing, it is stretched and often causes pain in the low back because of its direct pull on the inside of the lumbar vertebrae. Therefore, the iliopsoas muscle especially needs flexibility exercises.

Guidelines for Back Exercise

1. *Learn to distinguish between pain and discomfort.* When you have pain while exercising, that is a signal to stop. Some discomfort is to be expected and will go away shortly after the exercise is over. Don't exercise when pain is present.

2. *Progression should be slow.* If you are recovering from a back problem, allow yourself three to six months to achieve the strength and flexibility needed by your back to resist strains and sprains. In fact, you may not notice any improvement for a month or two. But don't give up. You're laying the foundations for future noticeable gains.

3. *Exercise every day.* When you first begin your back exercise program, since the number of repetitions will be so few, you need to exercise every day. After you achieve satisfactory levels of strength and flexibility, you can perform the exercises three days per week to maintain. The satisfactory level is achieved when you can perform the target goal of repetitions established for each exercise as stated in the previous chapter.

4. *Warm up before doing the exercise.* If your back has discomfort, take a short walk or take a warm bath or shower before doing the back exercises.

5. *Think positively.* Remind yourself that these exercises will work and that you will not give up. Commit yourself to do them every day until you achieve your goal.

Specific Exercises for Preventing Back Problems

Do the following exercises in the order listed below.

1. *Curl-up.* This was described in chapter 10 under the heading of "lead-up situp." Full situps should be avoided when you are recovering from a back problem. Begin by doing five repetitions. Add one or two repetitions each week. Your goal should be to do sixty without stopping.

After you have done sixty daily for at least a month, you can then begin to gradually replace curl-ups with situps. For example, do fifty-five curl-ups and five situps for two weeks. Then do fifty curl-ups and ten situps for two weeks. If no pain occurs during the situps, continue to increase them until all sixty are situps.

2. *Pelvic raises.* This exercise was described in chapter 10 under calisthenics. Begin as you did with the curl-up, starting at five and adding one or two each week until you are able to do sixty without stopping.

3. *Side leg raises.* This exercise was also described in chapter 10 under calisthenics. As with situps and pelvic raises, begin with five on each side the first week and add one or two each week until you are able to do forty without stopping.

4. *Knees to chest or low-back stretch.* This exercise was also described in the last chapter. Begin by doing three a day, then add one per week until you are able to do twenty. When just recovering from a back problem, you will feel discomfort in your back muscles. However, as your back heals and your flexibility increases, you will feel no discomfort in your back muscles during this exercise. As flexibility increases, reduce the repetitions to ten and add the next exercise.

5. *Hamstring stretch.* This exercise was described in chapter 10 under flexibility exercises. You should add this exercise only after you can perform the knees-to-chest with no discomfort. Start with three repetitions, hold for ten seconds, and add one per week until you reach ten repetitions.

6. *Quadriceps stretch.* This exercise was described in chapter 10 under flexibility exercises. Start with three repetitions, hold for ten seconds, and add one per week until you reach ten repetitions.

7. *Leg raises.* You should not start leg raises until you are free from pain and have advanced to twenty curl-ups a day. Begin by raising one leg at a time. From the regular lying position with both knees bent, straighten your left leg, keeping it flat on the floor. Slowly raise it, keeping the knee straight as high as you can. Then slowly lower it to the floor. Relax for a moment, and then repeat. Switch legs and repeat with the right leg. Begin by doing three with each leg, and add one or two each week until you are doing twenty.

After you are successfully doing twenty single-leg raises with no back pain, begin to do some leg raises with both legs together. First, do twenty with each leg separately and then do two with both legs together. Always do twenty single legs first, and then begin adding one or two double legs each week until you can do twenty single and twenty double.

8. *Back extensions.* This exercise was also explained in chapter 10 and should begin *only* after you are free from back pain. Begin by doing two and adding one each week until you can do fourteen.

9. *Donkey kicks.* This exercise was explained in chapter 10. Begin with three for each leg and increase one per week until you can do thirty for each leg.

10. *Hanging.* Whether you hang upright or inverted, hang thirty seconds to one minute each day. Most of the day you are either standing or sitting so your vertebrae are compressed. Hanging helps the vertebral column to elongate, which reduces the pressure on each vertebral disc. (Do not hang inverted if you have heart disease or high blood pressure.)

Sports and Activities

If you are really serious about overcoming a back problem, you will very closely monitor your other activities during your rehabilitation process. Jumping in basketball, twisting and bending in racquetball, arching your back in the tennis serve, rotating your trunk in golf, and the jarring of jogging are all hard on a lame back. Eliminate these activities and others like them until your back is free from pain and you have achieved the maximal goal for each back exercise. This may take three months to a year, but if you permanently overcome your back problem, it is well worth it. Don't think in terms of days or weeks but in terms of months and years. It's a lifestyle.

You don't, however, want to ignore your cardiorespiratory system. You need to continue an aerobic exercise program while rehabilitating your back. By far the best aerobic exercise for a person with back trouble is swimming. Swimming not only is good for the cardiorespiratory system but also is therapeutic for the back.

Another excellent aerobic exercise is cycling. Cycling indoors or outdoors to maintain your aerobic activity is also good for your back. Walking is usually recommended for a person with a bad back. As your back begins to heal, you can combine some jogging with your walking but listen to your back. If it bothers you, return to walking.

Other Lifestyle Factors

Several additional factors are crucial to preventing back problems. These include posture, lifting habits, weight reduction, and stress management.

Posture

Good posture is first of all a habit, and habits are formed by constant repetition. Second, good posture results from strong muscles, and strong muscles require a muscle-development exercise program. If we develop the habits and the muscles for good posture, we won't have as many back problems. Equally important, we will work more efficiently, look younger, and appear self-confident.

If there is one word that would best convey the mental image of good posture and body alignment, it would be *tall* (think tall). Adherence to the following three practices will lead to good posture:

1. Hold your head up high and tall. Feel as though you are trying to touch the ceiling with the top of your head.
2. Raise your chest, rib cage, and shoulders.
3. Tilt your pelvis backward by contracting your abdominal muscles and your gluteal muscles.

In addition to practicing good postural habits, when standing for long periods of time, you should place one foot on a stool, chair, or other object. You can alternate your feet to allow shifts of weight and still keep your back from excess sway, or *lordosis*. When sitting while reading, watching television, or studying, you should place your feet (with knees bent) on a stool or a footrest. The chair should have a good, firm seat with a cushion. Don't slump. The same advice should apply in driving a car; your knees should be bent. Move the seat of the car as close to the steering wheel as feasible to prevent swayback. It is also helpful on long trips to stop at rest areas that afford a table or bench and perform back exercises and stretching.

Lifting Habits

Improper lifting of heavy objects or carrying heavy objects can place considerable pressure on the vertebral column and lead to back problems. Thus, proper lifting technique is extremely important. When you lift objects from the floor, your knees should be bent so that the lifting is done with your legs rather than your back. When placing groceries into the trunk of a car, raising windows, hanging up clothes, cooking, making a bed, or reaching for objects, you should lift with the object as close to your body as possible. When you lift objects while turning, since there is less stability and support of the vertebrae, your feet and entire body should be rotated as a unit.

Weight Reduction

Excess weight, primarily fat, in addition to placing harmful pressures on the cardiovascular system and other systems of the body, also places undesirable stress on the vertebral column. The extra twenty or thirty pounds of weight often carried on the abdomen places considerable strain upon the back and can lead to back pain.

Stress Management

If a person is under constant stress, all the muscles in the body become tense. The slightest jar can cause a strain or sprain in a back muscle. Persons with low-back pain often have a recurrence when involved in a stressful situation. It is important to effectively manage the stress you face.

Steps You Could Take

1. Do you have any of the lifestyle habits that may contribute to back pain?
   a. Do you have good flexibility in the low-back muscles as evidenced by the sit-and-reach test?
   b. Do you have a strong abdomen as evidenced by meeting the standard for situps?
   c. Do you have good low-back and gluteal strength as evidenced by the back extension and pelvic raise tests?
   d. Do you have good posture?
   e. Do you lift objects carefully?
   f. Are you overweight?
   g. Are you tense?

2. Set a time aside three to five days each week when you will do the back exercises listed in this chapter.

12

The Physically Active Lifestyle

It is so easy to neglect the care of our bodies, especially our daily need to exercise and to have physical activity. This seems particularly true of Christians who find time daily to read the Bible and pray and who regularly attend church. We don't mean to neglect our bodies. We have good intentions to begin an exercise program. Many New Year's resolutions have been made, but as we get caught up in the hustle and bustle of each day, somehow the exercise time vanishes.

Regular Exercise Guidelines

Regular physical exercise is not a luxury. It is not an I'll-do-it-when-I-get-around-to-it proposition. Taking care of your body is your God-given responsibility. Remember, your body is God's temple, and it has been bought with a price. We encourage you to use the following guidelines to assist you in exercising regularly.

1. *Build into your daily and weekly schedule the time of day you are going to exercise and stick to it.* Determine what time of the day will best suit your schedule and lock in a time for exercise. It really doesn't matter whether it is morning, noon, or night. The best time is whatever time you can program into your daily schedule.

2. *Don't go by how you feel!* Many times I have come to my scheduled exercise periods with a tired feeling or a slight headache as the result of a busy day. The temptation is to lie down and rest. But I have learned that when I feel the least like exercising, that is precisely when I need it the most and will benefit the greatest. Don't let your feelings rule your intellect. Discipline your mind to do what is good for you regardless of your feelings.

Of course, to all guidelines there are exceptions. If you don't feel like exercising because of illness, especially when you have a fever, then listen to your body and rest it. But never skip an exercise session because of mental fatigue.

3. *Never ask yourself, Should I work out today?* This question is not a part of the active lifestyle. The only decision you have is *when*, not *should I?* If you ever let yourself ask this question, you might as well forget your exercise that day. You can always come up with a hundred excuses, all valid, about why you should not exercise. You probably don't ask yourself if you should brush your teeth or if you should eat each day. Daily exercise should also be a daily imperative.

4. *You can always do some form of exercise.* This guideline has two aspects. First, some injury may prevent your doing your normal exercise routine. You may normally be engaged in a walking/jogging program, but you injure your knee and can't walk or jog purposefully. Don't just sit there! Find some alternative exercise such as swimming or riding a bike. If you can't do either of those, double or triple your calisthenics until your knee is better. But do something to keep your muscles active.

Second, you may have a permanent disability that prevents your doing many exercises you would like to do. A student at ORU was in a car accident and broke his neck. He was paralyzed from the upper abdomen down. For more than a year he needed constant attention. He couldn't get in or out of a car unassisted, he had to be pushed in his wheelchair, and he could not get into and out of his wheelchair alone. But he had the same need everyone else does; he needed to exercise his muscles that weren't paralyzed. He needed to keep his heart strong, and he needed to keep his body from depositing fat.

We started him on a swimming program. At first, he was helped into and out of the water as well as assisted while in the water. The program was remarkably successful. The paralyzed muscles remained paralyzed, but the muscles in the remainder of his body strengthened to the point that a year later he was self-sufficient. He could get into and out of his wheelchair by himself, could move the wheelchair by himself, drive a car, and totally take care of himself. Everyone can do some form of exercise.

5. *Aerobic and back exercises are basic.* Regardless of the additional exercises you do, aerobic and back exercises must be a part of your regular activity program. I have no problem with my aerobic exercises. I faithfully jog, swim, or cycle five or six days per week, fifty-two weeks a year. But I find it easy to ignore the back exercises and have often paid the price for the neglect. I personally find it the easiest to discipline myself if I do the back exercises when I first get out of bed in the morning. I roll

onto the floor, eyes still half-shut, and do the back exercises before I'm fully awake. One, two...zzzzz...twenty...zzz...fifty. Now I'm awake and ready for the day. I do my aerobic exercises at noon or between 4:30 and 5:30 in the afternoon before dinner.

6. *You're never too busy to exercise.* How often do we use that for an excuse! "I just don't have time to exercise!" Actually, you don't have time *not* to exercise. C. James Krafft, M.D., former director of student health at Oral Roberts University, insists that he is so busy he can't afford to take less than one hour a day to exercise. Exercise gives you more vitality and energy so you'll have more vigor to do the remaining tasks.

Studies have shown that an exercise break enhances mental concentration following the exercise. Solutions to problems come faster. Both a judge in Tulsa and the president of one of the largest oil companies in America have told me that their late afternoon aerobics programs have become absolute necessities, not only for the physiological benefits but also for the psychological and relaxation benefits. Both men start their days at the office before 7:00 A.M. and often don't leave until after 6:00 P.M. But before they go home, rather than go to the club for a drink, they go for a two- to five-mile jog in the aerobics center. It wakes them up, burns off the stress and tension of the day, and prepares them for the evening that often involves more work.

7. *Get a new hairdo.* Many women protest they have difficulty crowding in an exercise session because it will take them too long to arrange their hair afterward. Perhaps they need to look at their priorities and decide what in life is more important: fancy hair or a healthy and physically fit body. I've never heard of someone getting sick and going to the hospital with hair problems, but I surely hear about health problems.

Up until Donna went to work, her time to exercise was ample as was time to arrange her hair. Working eight hours a day changed that. To her, keeping a healthy and trim body was the priority. So, short hair with a curly permanent was the way to manage her hair. Her daily schedule in the Student Health Clinic at ORU is 8:00 A.M. to 4:30 P.M., with an hour for lunch. The one hour is spent efficiently: 10 minutes—going to locker, changing into exercise clothing; 5 minutes—stretching for flexibility, doing warm-up and calisthenics; 25 minutes—jogging three miles; 10 minutes—showering and dressing; and 10 minutes—eating lunch (apple, sandwich, yogurt, carrot sticks).

8. *Get in shape to participate in sports; don't expect sports to get you in shape.* Many persons have the misconception that they will develop their personal health and fitness through a program of tennis, racquetball, basketball, or some other sport. In most cases this doesn't work. Even athletes don't expect that participating in the sport will get them in

shape. Coaches always have an off-season and preseason conditioning program during which time they get their players in shape to play the game. Health and fitness are the foundations upon which sports are played.

Aerobic exercises (walking/jogging, swimming, and cycling), back exercises, and muscle exercises (weight training and calisthenics) are the building blocks upon which sports skills can be built. Participating in the sport before developing fitness is like building a house upon the sand. Muscle soreness, joint pain, and other problems are likely to develop.

9. *You're never too old to exercise.* I recently asked a ninety-one-year-old woman at the Oral Roberts' retirement center, "What keeps you so young?" She has her own apartment, cooks some of her own meals, gives visitors tours of the center, and is full of enthusiasm and vigor. She said, "Never slow down!" She walks three miles every day, takes care of a small garden, and continues to keep her mind active.

Another woman at age seventy-eight had suffered two heart attacks and was so weak and feeble she spent most of her time in bed waiting to die. A daughter visited her and told her that another grandchild was on the way. She suggested her mother stay around a little longer to see it. The grandmother decided to try to get going again. She began to walk a few minutes three times a day, seven days per week. After two months she was walking fifteen minutes, three times a day. After six months she was walking thirty minutes, three times a day. After a year, it was three daily one-hour walks. She was beginning to feel so good that she thought she would try some jogging. At age eighty-four, six years after she first started, she was jogging five miles a day. She now has a strong heart. You're never too old to engage in regular exercise.

The Active Lifestyle

The regular exercise program consisting of aerobic exercises, back exercises, and other muscle-building exercises is going to take between thirty and ninety minutes per day, three to six times per week. For example, if you spent one hour per day, six days per week exercising, it would add up to six hours per week. Of the total 168 hours in a week, this would mean that 162 hours are spent not exercising. Therefore, while a sixty-minute total exercise session a day is highly beneficial and will markedly enhance your optimal health and fitness, you need to examine what you do the rest of the day.

Two persons can be involved in the same exercise program, but one may improve much faster than the other. Consider Tom and Bill as examples. Both enrolled in an adult fitness program at the same time, and both were of the same approximate age and initial fitness. Tom improved much faster than Bill, even though both were basically doing the same exercise routines. Why?

The answer could be found in what they were doing the rest of the week. Tom took his dog for a walk each night, worked several evenings a week in his big garden, kicked a soccer ball around with his kids, and every few weekends would go backpacking with friends. Bill spent his evenings and weekends playing the piano, working on his stamp collection, and watching television. Therefore, in addition to the regular exercise program, Tom was far more active in his regular day-to-day living than was Bill. Tom improved faster because his whole lifestyle was one of greater physical activity.

Look at your total life. Do you have an active lifestyle over and above your regular exercise program? Be conscious of exercise-saving devices and avoid them. Consider incorporating the following ideas into your lifestyle.

1. *Use the stairs rather than the elevator.* When you are given a choice at your place of work or a shopping center, use the stairs. You would be astonished in a month or year what a difference this one little lifestyle change makes.

2. *Park your car farther away from your destination.* Do you ever go shopping and park your car as close to the store as possible? Maybe even park where you're not supposed to? Try parking your car farther away from the store and walking. When you go to church, park your car away from the door and walk. Not only are you helping yourself to be more fit, you're leaving open parking spots closer to the door for handicapped persons and persons who need to park closer.

3. *Walk, don't ride.* Do you have friends who live within a mile of your house? What about a store? What about your place of employment? If you answered yes, walk to your friends' homes, walk to the store when you're purchasing only a small amount, and walk to work. Not only are you helping yourself to increase your fitness, you are conserving energy (gasoline) and saving yourself money.

4. *Develop hobbies that require physical effort.* This does not imply that sedentary hobbies are bad. However, if all your leisure-time pursuits are sedentary, you need to reexamine them. Have some hobbies that involve physical activity. Gardening, backpacking, boating, or participating in sports activities, such as tennis, golf, badminton, horseshoes, bowling, and many others, while not appreciably producing fitness, complement your regular exercise program.

5. *Emphasize sports participation, not sports spectatorship.* Many Amer-

ican males claim to be great sportsmen. Their sports activity involves reading the sports section of the paper and *Sports Illustrated* and watching football, baseball, basketball, and golf on TV or in person. Their personal sports and exercise program is zero. When this type of individual does decide to exercise, he goes all out on the weekend and is a physical wreck on Monday. He does himself more harm than good. Before you take up watching sports as a hobby, make sure you have your own personal exercise and sports program.

6. *Avoid labor-saving devices.* Of course, use a power mower to mow your lawn but use one you push, not one that can be ridden or is self-propelled. What about homemade ice cream? Hard to beat occasionally. But don't use an electric motor to churn it. Buy an ice-cream maker you crank yourself. Automatic remote control for your TV? Forget it! Get up out of the chair and walk to the TV when you want to change channels. Play golf. It's a fine sport for recreation which can complement your regular exercise program. But don't use a golf cart. If you play eighteen holes, you could walk five miles.

Physical-activity-related Injuries

We would like to close our eyes to this fact, but injuries occasionally occur as a result of physical activity programs. The majority of injuries usually occur early in a physical activity program when a person may be progressing too rapidly. However, most persons who engage in a serious exercise program for any length of time eventually suffer some form of injury. The injury is usually a minor one that disappears within a few days. "An ounce of prevention is worth a pound of cure" is an applicable adage in discussing injuries.

Throughout this book certain guidelines of conditioning have been described. If you follow them, not only will you improve your fitness, but you will have fewer injuries. It is not possible to list every exercise injury, but the following ones are fairly common.

Blisters

A blister occurs when fluid fills the area between the dermis and the epidermis of the skin. The basic *cause* is excess heat to the skin as a result of friction. The friction is often related to shoes that fit improperly, wrinkled socks, or new shoes that are not broken in.

The best *prevention* for blisters is to buy shoes that fit properly. If shoes are too short, they will crowd the toes and cause blisters in the toes. The shoe should be one-quarter- to one-half-inch longer than the big toe. The width should allow movement of all toes. Wear two pairs of socks and don't let them wrinkle.

If you feel an area of heat, called a "hot spot," developing, stop the activity immediately. Apply cold water or ice to the skin at the site of the hot spot in order to cool it down and prevent the blister from forming. You may also apply petroleum jelly to spots where blisters tend to form.

As for *treatment*, if the blister is small, cover it with first-aid cream, gauze, and tape, leaving the tape on for four to six days. If the blister is large and hurts, puncture it with a sterilized needle, squeeze the fluid out, cover it with first-aid cream, gauze, and tape. A "donut" may be made from gauze and applied around the blister to prevent further friction to the area. You might also check with your local pharmacy about a spray that may be applied to the skin to temporarily toughen it. This is great for backpackers. Also, a product called "Second Skin" may be applied over the blister.

Muscle Soreness

The precise cause of muscle soreness is not known; however, it is probably due to two reasons. First, the muscles may feel stiff and swollen because of an accumulation of metabolic waste products that have not yet been removed. Second, minute tears in muscle fibers or connective tissue may cause the pain. The basic *cause* of muscle soreness is participation in unaccustomed exercise, which may be a new exercise, sudden movements, or a muscle worked harder than it is used to. It is natural to feel some general soreness four to eight hours after an exercise, and it may last twenty-four to forty-eight hours. Any soreness beyond forty-eight hours, however, indicates excessive muscle soreness; the activity you engaged in was too strenuous.

The best *prevention* for muscle soreness is to warm up before an activity and then follow a program of gradual progression. *Treatment* for muscle soreness is resting the muscles, applying ice for the first twenty-four hours, and then heating and stretching out the sore muscles. You can continue to exercise with a sore muscle because this will not further injure it. However, the exercise should be light.

Shin Splints

One very common type of muscle strain, especially for new joggers, is shin splints. Shin splints cause pain on either side of the shin bone (front of the lower leg), and the pain is increased by pointing the toes toward the floor or toward the shin. The *causes* of shin splints are numerous, including having fallen arches, overusing muscles, running on hard surfaces, not warming up with stretching exercises for the shin and back leg area, wearing shoes that lack a good arch support or have poorly cushioned soles, and running improperly. Probably the primary cause of shin splints is running faster and farther than you are normally able to, that is, progressing too rapidly. Careful avoidance of these causes is the best *prevention* of shin splints.

Shin splints are either acute or chronic. Acute shin splints are painful during the exercise, but the pain leaves when the exercise is over. This is not a cause for serious concern. When shin splints become chronic, however, you feel pain not only when you jog but also when you walk slowly. If you continue to run at a pace with the pain, the muscle tears will increase until the muscle is actually tearing away from the shinbone. Permanent scar-tissue damage can result.

The primary *treatment* for acute shin splints is to slow down your jogging pace, rest more days in between jogging, warm up longer, wear good shoes, and prevent your acute shin splints from becoming chronic. To treat chronic shin splints, rest (*no jogging*), apply heat or ice to the area, buy shoes with good arch supports, and stretch out the muscles well. Use an alternative exercise such as cycling or swimming.

Sprain

A sprain is an injury to a ligament which is either stretched or torn. The function of ligaments is to prevent bones from separating and moving beyond the normal range of motion. Sprains particularly occur to the ligaments that make up joints in the ankle and knee. When a ligament in your ankle is stretched because you step in a hole or turn your foot in, your ankle is sprained. You will then experience pain and swelling in that area.

The ligament is not made of materials that will stretch and return to its normal length as readily as will its counterpart, the muscle. Thus, once you have sprained or stretched a ligament, it is not likely to return to its normal length. Therefore, preventing ligaments from being sprained is of utmost importance. One of the best ways of *prevention* is to strengthen the muscles that support the knee joint, namely, the hamstring and quadriceps muscle groups. If the muscles are strong, they can help hold the bones of the joints in place so that the ligaments are not injured.

The best *treatment* for a sprain is threefold. Elevate the injured part, apply ice for twenty minutes every four hours (up to twenty-four to thirty-six hours), and wrap it to compress it. After twenty-four to thirty-six hours, you can apply heat. You should immobilize it as much as possible for one to two weeks after which you should begin conditioning exercises to strengthen the muscles around the joint.

Side Ache

A side ache is a pain, sometimes dull and sometimes sharp, which usually but not always occurs in the right side. It is common to conditioned and nonconditioned athletes alike. A side ache is not an injury or a ruptured appendix. Every person will probably at one time or another experience it.

Several theories exist as to the *cause* of a side ache. It is commonly believed to be a spasm caused by an insufficient oxygen supply to the diaphragm muscle. The basic *prevention* of a side ache is to avoid exercising beyond the overload you are capable of handling at a particular time. The better your condition, the more oxygen will be supplied to the diaphragm muscle and the fewer side aches you will have. Activities too soon after a meal may also precipitate a side ache. Weak abdominal muscles have been considered a factor in causing side aches, as have inadequate warm-ups. The *treatment* for a side ache is normally to slow down whatever activity you are doing. Then the pain will usually go away.

Joint Injuries

Injuries to the joints are possible with any physical activity, especially jogging. Trauma and jarring of the joints, especially the knee and hip joints, are experienced in jogging. By jogging on soft surfaces and wearing a pair of good shoes with thick soles, you can work toward *prevention* of joint injuries. The best *treatment* for joint injuries is rest. If you have pain in a joint while jogging, stop jogging. Do an alternate form of activity, such as cycling or swimming, and allow the joint to heal. Continued jogging on an injured joint will only aggravate the injury and prevent healing. You must rest a joint in order for it to heal and then gradually progress back into a jogging program.

Ice Treatment

The immediate treatment for virtually any type of injury, especially sprains, joint injuries, and bruises, is ice. The purpose of ice treatment is to reduce the swelling by constricting the blood vessels, thus decreasing the bleeding in the area of the injury. The ice treatment should last ten to twenty minutes and can be repeated every four hours for twenty-four to thirty-six hours after the injury. After this period, heat can be applied to the injury since the bleeding should have stopped. Ice treatment takes two forms—ice immersion and ice pack.

1. *Ice immersion.* This is useful if the injury is to the foot, ankle, lower leg, hand, wrist, or arm. Fill a pail or tub with cold tap water. Place the

injured part in the water. As the injured area becomes accustomed to the cold, gradually add ice to the water. Keep it in the ice water for ten to twenty minutes. Remove the injured part, dry it off, elevate it for ten minutes, and lightly wrap it with an elastic wrap. Repeat this every four hours for twenty-four to thirty-six hours.

2. *Ice pack.* When the injured area, such as the upper leg or back, would be too difficult to immerse in ice water, an ice pack can be placed on it. Place a half gallon of crushed ice in an ice bag or in a plastic sack (a double-thick bread sack works well). Wrap a towel around the sack, and place the sack directly on the injury. If possible, wrap the ice pack to the injury in order to ensure good, close contact of the ice and the injured part. Leave the pack on for ten to twenty minutes; then follow the same process as the ice immersion.

Prayer

In addition to the application of the natural laws to assist in a speedy recovery from any injury, apply the spiritual principles discussed in chapter 3. What power Christians have when they apply both natural and spiritual laws of God's creation!

Steps You Could Take

The physically active lifestyle that will truly result in a high degree of health and fitness is more than just a regular exercise program. It involves a conscious effort on your part to be physically active as much of the day as possible.

1. Examine your lifestyle and explore ways of being more active.

2. If you jog or walk, make sure you have a *good* pair of jogging shoes.

3. Progress slowly in your exercise program to prevent injuries.

Part III

Body Composition and Nutritional Health

13

Understanding Body Composition

Body Composition

Most of us are concerned about our weight. We often go on diets to lose weight. We compare our weight to height-weight charts to see if we are overweight. We associate overweight with fat. In reality, body weight is not as important as body composition. Body composition evaluates how much of your weight is fat.

Your body weight is made up of four major components: bone, muscle, body organs, and fat. The weights of your bones and, to a large degree, your body organs are set by heredity, and you cannot control them. Some people have big bones and some have small bones. The size of your bones is of no consequence for health. But you do control the weight of your body that is made up of muscle and fat. The average adult male and female have the approximate body compositions noted in the following table.

TABLE 13.1
Average Adult Body Composition

BODY COMPONENT	MALE		FEMALE	
	WEIGHT (LB.)	PERCENT	WEIGHT (LB.)	PERCENT
Bone	25.5	15	15.6	12
Muscle	68.0	40	42.9	33
Body organs	42.5	25	32.5	25
Fat	34.0	20	39.0	30
Total	170.0	100	130.0	100

That the average male has 20 percent of his weight made up of fat and the average female has 30 percent of her weight made up of fat doesn't mean the percentage is acceptable. In fact, the average person has too high a percentage of fat on the body. With the excess fat come numerous health problems that will be discussed in chapter 14.

Fat Versus Muscle

Weight alone is not a good measure of body composition since we don't know how much of the weight is fat and how much is muscle. Excess muscle weight is healthful; excess fat weight is unhealthful. Therefore, in addition to weight we should also measure fat. In our testing at Oral Roberts University we often find persons of the same height and weight with considerably different body fat percentages. For instance, we may measure two girls (Susan and Jill) who are both five feet six inches tall and weigh 130 pounds. One may have 35 percent fat, and the other may have only 20 percent. Both weigh 130, but their body compositions would be different as the following table shows.

TABLE 13.2
Body Composition Comparisons

BODY COMPONENT	SUSAN WEIGHT (LB.)	PERCENT	JILL WEIGHT (LB.)	PERCENT
Bone	15.6	12	15.6	12
Muscle	36.4	28	55.9	43
Body organs	32.5	25	32.5	25
Fat	45.5	35	26.0	20
Total	130.0	100	130.0	100

Both girls have the same weight in bones and body organs, but of the total body weight of 130 pounds, Susan has 36.4 pounds of muscle and 45.5 pounds of fat and Jill has 55.9 pounds of muscle and only 26 pounds of fat. Jill enjoys greater optimal health than Susan. She also has a smaller dress size (size eight) compared to Susan's dress size (size twelve). As we shall see, that didn't happen by chance.

In chapter 11, I described a man who stopped all exercise for three months to recover from a slipped disc. During this time, his weight remained the same—160 pounds. His body fat, however, increased from 13 percent to 17 percent, a 4 percent increase in fat or 6.8 pounds. In order for him to gain 6.8 pounds of fat but have his total body weight stay the same, he also lost 6.8 pounds of muscle during this sedentary period, obviously a negative change.

This is what occurs with age in typical sedentary persons. Their weights may stay about the same, but their body compositions change. They may lose muscle and gain fat. (Please note that muscle does not turn to fat. Rather, muscle tissue atrophies and fat tissue enlarges.) Former President Ford is a prime example. He stated that as president he was the same weight he was when he played college football. However, his slack size had increased from a thirty-four-inch waist to a thirty-eight-inch waist. Something had happened to his body composition in forty years. That does not have to happen! If you maintain an active lifestyle and perform your aerobic exercises and your muscle-building exercises, you can keep the muscles and keep off the fat.

How Much Fat Is Acceptable?

The acceptable percentage of fat on your body for good health is outlined in Table 13.3.

TABLE 13.3
Body Fat Standards

HEALTH FITNESS STANDARDS	MALES (%)	FEMALES (%)
Lean	5–10	10–20
Excellent	10–15	20–25
Acceptable	15–20	25–30
Overfat	20–25	30–35
Obese	25 plus	35 plus

Some fat on the body is absolutely essential for health. Males should have at least 5 percent and females at least 10 percent to 15 percent fat unless they are highly conditioned athletes and in competition.

Recently Dr. Tom Bassler, a pathologist, reported his results of autopsies conducted on several highly trained male long-distance runners who died from apparent heart attacks. His conclusion was that they didn't die from a normal heart attack. Their coronary arteries were healthy with little or no atherosclerosis. Rather, they died from a cardiac arrhythmia that was triggered by a combination of three factors: (1) their body fat was less than 5 percent, (2) they had been jogging more than eighty to one hundred miles per week, and (3) they were on a restricted diet that prevented their receiving all the nutrients they needed. Each of these three factors alone is not a potential killer. However, when combined for a period of time they can be deadly.

When a female drops below 10 percent to 15 percent fat, she will quit having her menstrual period. Why this happens is not fully understood, but it may be the result of the decreased fat percentage throwing off the hormone levels of the body. Whether or not ovulation continues is also uncertain.

For health, an excellent amount of body fat for males appears to be 10 percent to 15 percent and for females 20 percent to 25 percent. A male whose body fat exceeds 25 percent and a female whose body fat exceeds 35 percent run the risk of numerous health problems. It really doesn't matter how much they weigh or whether they appear fat.

I have seen and tested football players who weigh 250 pounds and appear to be obese, but when their body fat is measured, they may have only 15 percent fat. The excess weight is all muscle. On the other hand, I have seen a six-foot-tall man who weighs 170 pounds and does not appear overweight; yet he has 25 percent fat and is actually obese according to body fat standards. He has very little muscle on his body.

How Is Body Fat Measured?

We have emphasized in this chapter that what you weigh is not very important, but body-fat percentage is highly important for health. Body fat can be measured, and you can learn to measure your own.

Body fat can be measured in two ways. We know that fat floats and muscle sinks. The overfat person can float in a pool more easily than a muscular person. Research laboratories have used this principle to measure a person's body fat. A chair is hung from a large scale and is placed in a tank of water. The subject sits in the chair, and while he is completely immersed in the water, his weight is taken. The more fat he has, the more he will float and the less he will weigh in water. The more muscle he has, the more he will sink and the more he will weigh. From the underwater weight measurement, several calculations can be made and the percentage of fat can be determined.

Although this procedure is accurate, it is obviously limited to the laboratory situation and won't help to determine your percentage of fat. Therefore, researchers have developed a "skinfold" method, which is a fairly accurate procedure and will estimate the percentage of fat within 1 percent or 2 percent of the actual underwater test.

A skinfold is a pinch of skin and fat. The thumb and forefinger pinch the skin so that the skinfold pinch should be made up of two layers of skin and the fat that lies just below the skin, but not the muscle. A specially designed caliper is placed approximately one centimeter (0.39 inch) from the fingers, and the thickness of the skinfold is measured. Since about 50 percent of the total body fat is located just beneath the skin, the thickness of the skinfold estimates total body fat.

The prediction of percentage of fat from skinfolds involves taking skinfold measurements at three or four body sites: usually the back of the arm, the abdomen, and several other designated areas. The skinfold thicknesses are combined, and the percentage of fat is determined. It is a simple process, but a caliper and directions are essential to measure your body fat.

Your physician may be able to make this measurement for you. (Unfortunately, very few do.) Or if there is a college or university near you, you could consult its health and physical education department to determine if it performs this procedure. Or, you could consult the YMCA or YWCA if one is nearby.

Steps You Could Take

1. Have your percentage of fat calculated. _____ Percentage of Fat. _____ Date

2. What is the health fitness standard of your body fat? _____

14

Obesity: Problems and Causes

It is a sad commentary on our way of life, but coupled with our lack of exercise, most Americans are eating themselves to death. More than half our population has excess body fat and suffers the resulting health problems. A young couple marry and the wife unknowingly sets out to kill her husband by the way she feeds him. Newly marrieds usually gain ten to twenty pounds of weight in the first two years of marriage, and the added weight is all fat.

We stated in the last chapter that some fat on the body is absolutely essential for health. But excess body fat serves no desirable purpose and leads to numerous health problems. The excess fat is "dead" weight, puts an added strain on the heart and circulatory system, has a detrimental effect on all body organs, and disrupts the normal hormone functions.

Health Problems Related to Excess Body Fat

Statistics clearly reveal that as body fat begins to exceed 25 percent for men and 35 percent for women, the death rate from numerous diseases increases. Life expectancy for the obese person is considerably shorter than for the normal person.

Some of the specific health problems associated with excess body fat are diseases of the heart and blood vessels. More heart attacks are suffered by obese persons. They also have higher blood pressure, greater atherosclerosis, more strokes, and elevated blood fats.

Diseases are not limited to the cardiovascular system. Obesity is considered the single most important factor in the cause of gallbladder disease. Excess body fat significantly contributes to diabetes and is associated with gout. Recent studies reveal a relationship between obesity and several types of cancer. Chances of complications during surgery and pregnancy are much greater in the obese person.

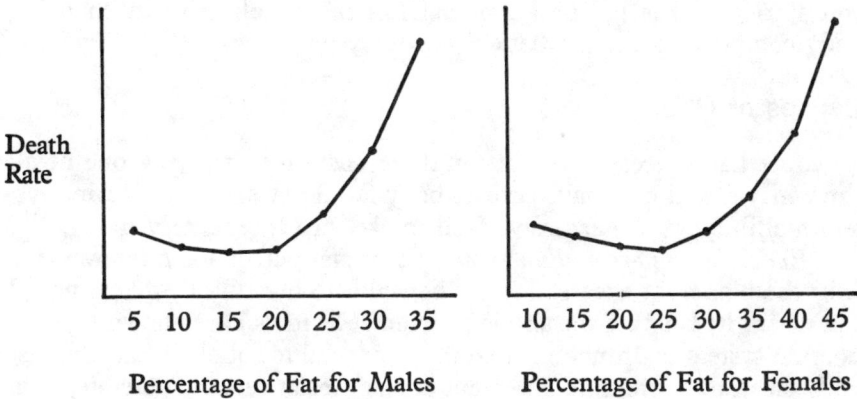

Death
Rate

| 5 10 15 20 25 30 35 | 10 15 20 25 30 35 40 45 |

Percentage of Fat for Males   Percentage of Fat for Females

Fig. 14.1. Death Rate in Relation to Percentage of Body Fat

Excess body fat is also related to orthopedic problems. Arthritis, rheumatism, and joint pain are far more common in the obese person. Mobility is a problem because of the excess fat. Studies show the overfat person is sick more often and misses as many as five times more days of work in a year than a person of normal weight.

Emotional and social problems also plague obese persons. They often feel embarrassed, guilty, and frustrated, and they have a low self-esteem.

God's Attitude Toward Excess Fat

We were created by God to function with a body composition that has approximately 5 percent to 20 percent fat and 40 percent to 55 percent muscle for men and 15 percent to 30 percent fat and 30 percent to 45 percent muscle for women. When body composition deviates too much from this range, there is an imbalance within the body. Disharmony develops among the body cells and organs, and disease results. *God did not create us to be fat!*

As we noted earlier, the Scriptures equate excess eating resulting in obesity (gluttony) with excess drinking of alcohol (drunkenness). Christians have generally been in agreement on the sin of drunkenness, but they have overlooked the sin of gluttony. God doesn't. "Do not mix with winebibbers,/ Or with gluttonous eaters of meat;/ For the drunkard and the glutton will come to poverty" (Prov. 23:20–21).

It is not our purpose to condemn you if you are struggling with excess body fat. Perhaps you have tried many approaches to losing your fat. We'll reveal some of the reasons people become fat, and then we'll give you a tried and tested program that has proven effective in changing body composition for the better.

Causes of Obesity

People have excess body fat for three basic reasons. Any one or all three may function to cause excess body fat. They are (1) endocrine-system malfunction, (2) excessive food intake, or (3) sedentary living.

1. *Endocrine-system malfunction.* The overfat person too often wants to shift the blame for excess fat from behavior to heredity by declaring, "I can't help it; I have a metabolic problem." Studies have shown that endocrine-system malfunctions that upset normal metabolism cause excess body fat in no more than 5 percent of the overfat cases. Therefore, in at least 95 percent of overfat cases, the cause is not faulty metabolism but personal excesses. But since an endocrine-system malfunction is always a possibility, you should have a thorough physical examination by your physician to confirm or rule out this case. If your obesity has a partial root in an endocrine-system malfunction, taking medicine alone won't solve the problem. You still need to change your lifestyle in regard to diet and exercises to control your excess fat.

2. *Excessive food intake.* Some persons exercise more or less regularly and still have excess fat. If their exercise schedule is adequate for maintaining good body fat, then they must have a habit, a lifestyle of heavy eating, that offsets the exercise program.

The housewife, without realizing it, may be nibbling on food and snacks all day, sampling her cooking. Perhaps a businessman has numerous meetings over big breakfasts, luncheons, or dinners, and he is eating more than he realizes. Perhaps a youth loads up on junk food that is high in calories. Many people have a habit of eating too much in the evening while watching TV.

Overeating can also be due to emotional reasons. Some persons turn to food as a tranquilizer. When faced with loneliness, emergencies, difficult situations, homesickness, breakup of a romance, fear, anxiety, or numerous other stressful situations, these persons turn to food to find release from their problems.

If you are overfat, evaluate your eating habits and your motivation. If you conclude that your excess fat is simply due to a habit of eating too much and not to eating in response to situations, chapter 17 outlines an approach for helping you to control your eating habits. If your excessive eating is due to stressful circumstances, develop positive behaviors to manage your stress (see chaps. 18 and 19). If you have difficulty changing this lifestyle, consult a competent Christian counselor to receive assistance in overcoming the inner problem that leads to such behavior.

3. *Sedentary living.* The vast majority of persons with excess fat have gained it not because of a metabolic problem or because of excessive eating but because of sedentary living. Sedentary living is the cause in approximately 70 percent to 80 percent of obese persons. After years of being inactive and not following an aerobics program as outlined in chapters 8 and 9 and muscle exercises as outlined in chapters 10 and 11, the fat person's body composition has changed. When your body composition changes from less muscle to more fat, your entire internal body chemistry changes.

If two persons eat the same number of calories, persons with more fat on their bodies and less muscle will tend to store the calories in the food as body fat and gain weight. On the other hand, persons with more muscle on their bodies and less fat will tend to burn the calories in the food for energy and will not gain weight. Muscle tissue burns far more calories than fat tissue; therefore, a muscular person can eat more calories per day than a fat person.

So, most overfat persons are not that way because they eat too much. In fact, in many cases they eat less than persons of normal weight. The problem is that they have too little muscle to burn the calories they eat and they store the calories in fat. In these cases, the *only cure to obesity is regular exercise, not diet.*

Energy Balance

In order to maintain your weight, you must have a balance between your energy intake and your energy expenditure. Energy intake comes into the body in the form of all the foods we eat and liquids we drink, and we measure this in terms of calories. Some examples of the various caloric content of selected foods can be seen in the following table.

TABLE 14.1
Caloric Content of Selected Foods

FOOD	PORTION	CALORIES
Whole milk	1 cup	150
Skim milk	1 cup	85
Regular chocolate milk	1 cup	210
Apple juice	1 cup	120
Orange juice	1 cup	120
Soft drink	12 oz. can	145

FOOD	PORTION	CALORIES
Apple	1 medium size	80
Orange	1 medium size	65
Chocolate candy bar	1 normal size	300
Apple pie	1 piece	345
Pecan pie	1 piece	495
Whole wheat bread	1 piece	65
Peas	1 cup	77

The types of foods we eat make a tremendous difference in the calories we consume. A simple choice of drinking skim milk rather than whole milk can save you 65 calories per cup. If you drink three cups per day, you save 195 calories per day, which in a year translate into 71,175 calories. Since 3,500 calories is the equivalent of one pound of fat, this small choice in one year can help you lose twenty pounds.

Energy is expended by the body in three ways: (1) basal metabolic rate, (2) specific dynamic action (thermogenesis), and (3) physical activity.

1. *Basal Metabolic Rate (BMR)*. Your basal metabolic rate is the amount of energy required to continue all your body's basic functions at a resting level. It has long been accepted that your BMR, after age thirty, decreases at the rate of 0.5 percent per year. Therefore, since your body needs less energy to function at rest, you will gradually gain weight as you grow older if you continue to eat at the same level.

However, it has recently been discovered that your BMR doesn't automatically decrease with age, but rather it decreases in proportion to your muscle mass. Ansel Keys from the University of Minnesota reported only a 1 percent decrease in thirty years in physically active people. If you are inactive, you will lose muscle tissue and gain fat tissue as you grow older. Since muscle tissue demands more energy to stay alive than fat tissue, a decrease in muscle will automatically lower your BMR. If, on the other hand, you continue with an exercise program throughout your life, you will retain your muscle mass, and your BMR will go down only slightly.

The amount of energy necessary for BMR can be estimated for each thirty-year-old adult on the basis of the following equations. (These equations are only estimates for persons with normal metabolism and body composition. A person with less muscle and more fat, the BMR will be lower.)

Adult Men
BMR (calories) = add a zero to your weight + 2 times weight
Example: If a man weighs 150 pounds
Then, BMR (calories) = 1500
$$\underline{300}$$
1800 calories

Adult Women
BMR (calories) = add a zero to your weight + weight
Example: If a woman weighs 120 pounds
Then, BMR (calories) = 1200
$$\underline{120}$$
1320 calories

In these two examples, the amount of calories needed by the body per day is 1800 calories for the man and 1320 calories for the woman. This energy expenditure is needed to keep you alive.

2. *Specific dynamic action.* Specific dynamic action refers to the energy the body expends to digest food and to maintain normal body temperatures. This process includes churning the food in the stomach, moving it along the small intestine, absorbing it into the blood, and delivering it to the cells of the body. This requires only a small amount of energy, about 200 calories for men and 120 calories for women.

3. *Physical activity.* The third way we expend energy is through physical activity, not just the exercise type but also the activity of everyday living. Depending upon the level of physical activity, we can burn a considerable amount of calories through our daily activities.

Since energy expenditure from the BMR and the specific dynamic action routes is fairly stable, the greatest way to increase energy expenditure is through physical activity.

The person who wants to gain weight needs to consume more calories than he expends. The person who wants to lose weight must expend more calories than he consumes. If a male is expending 2150 calories per day and consuming 2650 calories, he has a *positive* balance of 500 calories. In seven days that positive balance will reach 3500 calories which will mean a one pound *weight gain*.

TABLE 14.2
Calories Expended Through Daily Physical Activity

LEVEL OF ACTIVITY	MEN	WOMEN
Sedentary—a person who performs daily tasks that require little physical activity, such as an office worker	150–225	125–200
Moderate—a person who engages in daily in 30-60 minutes of aerobic exercises	225–700	200–450
Heavy—a person who engages daily in 1-2 hours of aerobic activity	700 plus	450 plus

On the other hand, if the person expends 2150 calories per day and consumes only 1650 calories, he has a *negative* balance of 500 calories. Since he needs 500 more calories for energy than he is consuming, he will draw those calories from the stored fat in his body. Therefore, in seven days the negative balance will reach 3500 calories which will mean a one pound *weight loss*.

TABLE 14.3
Energy Expenditure Summary

SOURCE	MALE (150 LBS.)	FEMALE (120 LBS.)
BMR	1800	1320
Specific dynamic action	200	120
Physical activity	150–700+	125–450+
Total daily energy expenditure	2150–2850+	1565–2015+

Set-point Theory

Recently much has been written about the set-point theory, which basically states that your body weight (or more precisely, your body fat) is programmed to be at a "set point" and that your metabolism and eating habits will subconsciously work together to maintain that weight. I believe the set-point theory has some validity, but it can also be misleading.

People do have different metabolic rates. Two persons can eat the same amount of calories and have the same caloric expenditures, but one may lose weight and the other may actually gain. Therefore, every person must consume calories that correspond to his or her own metabolism.

However, to accept that we are destined by our set point to be at a certain body weight is inconsistent with physiology of exercise and nutrition as well as experience. I have seen scores of persons lose great amounts of weight and keep it off as a result of a complete lifestyle change. On the other hand, I have also seen many lose much weight only to gain it all back. The second group of persons tends to give credence to the set-point theory. That is, they regained the weight because of their set point.

However, the overwhelming evidence is that the persons regained their weight because they hadn't permanently changed their lifestyles. You can control your own weight through a total lifestyle of good exercise and dietary habits. "I can do all things through Christ who strengthens me" (Phil. 4:13).

Anorexia Nervosa

An opposite extreme to excessive eating is anorexia nervosa. Persons with this psychological disorder become so preoccupied with being thin and having no fat that they do not eat. This disorder is appearing with increased frequency in teen-age girls. No matter how thin the individuals, they still see themselves as fat. Unless this disorder is properly treated and corrected, the persons may literally starve to death. The person may eat large amounts of food, but then force themselves to throw up (bulimia). Anyone with this eating disorder needs professional counseling.

Steps You Could Take

1. If your body fat is more than 20 percent (men) or 30 percent (women), what is the primary cause? Overeating, sedentary living, or both?

2. What specific changes will you make to lower your percentage of fat?

3. If your body fat is below 5 percent (ment) or 10 percent (women) and you struggle with anorexia nervosa, what specific changes will you make to increase your weight and body fat?

4. Calculate your BMR and add to it your calories expended daily for specific dynamic action (SDA) and physical activity (PA).
   BMR _____
   SDA _____
   PS _____
   Total _____ calories/day

15

Shedding the Excess Fat

In the last chapter we noted that excess fat on the body is caused primarily by a lack of physical activity. This lack leads to a wasting away of muscle tissue (atrophy) and the expansion of body fat. Therefore, the primary method for treatment and prevention of excess body fat is a significant amount of exercise to develop muscle and burn fat.

Diets Alone Don't Work

Many persons develop a tremendous amount of self-discipline and try all kinds of fad diets. Some people consume only grapefruit, some just pineapples, and some only liquid protein drinks. Some people have fasted for weeks. On such diets you may lose some weight; in fact, you may lose a considerable amount of weight. But you don't lose much fat, you haven't developed muscle, and you haven't changed your body chemistry so the tendency to become fat is still present. In fact the body, deprived of food, increases its ability to store fat when the diet is over.

You can't pick up a popular magazine without reading about some new diet. The truth is, diet alone does not solve the problem of excess fat. It does not change the tendency to accumulate fat. Many diets are dangerous: they do not provide the body with the balanced nutrients it needs, and they are toxic to the body. Moreover, the primary body weight loss is water.

Some people say they will do anything to lose their excess fat. But they are often unwilling to do the one thing that can permanently solve the problem—exercise and stick with it.

Why Exercise?

To lose body fat you must first of all increase the functioning of the muscles on your body. As you begin exercising, your muscle mass will increase. This will increase your metabolism so that you are burning more of the calories you eat and your muscles will become more proficient in burning fat. That is why the muscular person can eat more food than the overfat person and still not gain weight. The increased metabolism burns more calories not only when you're exercising but even when you're sleeping. Also, fat is an insulator. The less fat you have, the more heat escapes from your body and the more energy your body must expend to maintain your 98.6-degree body temperature.

In chapter 13 we compared Susan and Jill. Both girls weigh the same—130 pounds—but because Jill has almost 20 pounds more muscle, she can eat approximately five hundred calories more per day than Susan and not gain weight! She can not only eat more, have the same weight, and have more muscle and less fat, but she will wear smaller dress sizes. Her waist, hips, and thighs will all be smaller because, pound-for-pound, muscle takes up less space than fat. Jill, however, didn't achieve a better-looking and healthier body composition by wishing or dieting alone. It was the result of exercise. Muscle develops only in response to exercise. Excess fat is burned only as a result of sustained exercise.

The Aerobics Exercise Program for Fat Loss

The exercise program for the overfat person will basically be the same as for everyone but with a couple of modifications. In chapter 8, the guidelines and progressions for an aerobic exercise program were aimed at developing cardiorespiratory fitness and burning fat. The guidelines listed were for persons of normal body composition. If you fall in the obese category (over 25 percent fat for men and over 35 percent for women), some modifications in the heart-rate intensity and duration must be followed.

When we are at rest, regardless of our body fat, the energy for our muscles to function comes two-thirds from burning fats and one-third from burning carbohydrates. When we begin to exercise mildly (55 percent to 65 percent maximum heart rate), we continue at the same ratio— two-thirds fat, one-third carbohydrates. After approximately 65 percent intensity, the fit and the unfit persons' metabolisms begin to differ. The fit person will continue to burn two-thirds fat and one-third carbohydrates until the intensity is 85 percent to 95 percent maximum. Some outstanding marathon runners continue to burn primarily fat up to 95 percent maximum. At that point, they begin to burn more carbohydrates than fat.

The unfit person begins to switch from burning fat to burning more carbohydrates at a much lower intensity. As the intensity increases from 70 percent to 80 percent, the unfit person will burn almost 90 percent carbohydrates for energy. If you are trying to lose body fat, that is exactly what you don't want to happen. This defeats the whole purpose of the exercise. You want to burn primarily fat, not carbohydrates, in order to lose body fat.

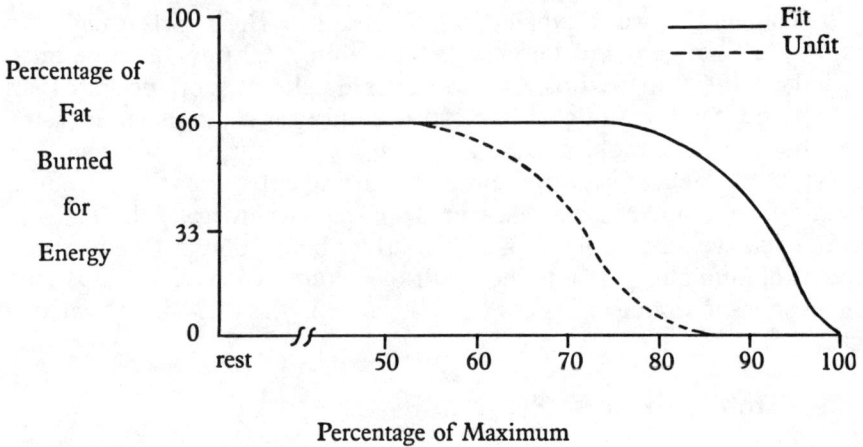

Percentage of Maximum

When you begin to burn primarily carbohydrates, in addition to not burning fat, several other negative events are occurring. Waste products are building up that quickly lead to pain and exhaustion. You may also have low blood sugar (*hypoglycemia*) that will trigger hunger and lead to eating. Therefore, you must keep the aerobic exercise intensity at 55 percent to 65 percent of your maximal heart rate and exercise for a longer duration.

You will note that the duration is longer than that outlined in chapter 8. You build up to seventy-five minutes. And you do this six days per week, nothing less. The overfat person must increase the duration in order for the fat to be burned off. If your duration is shorter, it takes longer to lose the fat. It is an extra price to pay in time, but the benefits are worthwhile.

TABLE 15.1
Progression Rate 5*
For a Person with Excess Body Fat

WEEK	HEART-RATE INTENSITY (%)	DURATION IN MINUTES
1	55	20
2	55	25
3	55	30
4	55	35
5	55	40
6	55	45
7	55–65	45
8	55–65	50
9	55–65	55
10	55–65	60
11	55–65	65
12	55–65	70
13	55–65	75
14	65	65
15	65	70
16	65	75
17	65–75	60
18	65–75	65
19	65–75	70
20	65–75	75
21	75	60
22	75	65
23	75	70
24	75	75

25th week and thereafter—continue at this intensity and duration until your percentage of fat is below 20 percent for men and 30 percent for women. Then you can follow the exercise combinations found in chapter 8.

*A progression for aerobic exercise for the person who needs to lose body fat. Based upon 6 days per week of walking, cycling, and/or swimming.

Once you achieve seventy-five minutes at 75 percent heart-rate intensity, continue at that level until your percentage of fat is below 20 percent for men and 30 percent for women. When that occurs you can increase your intensity and shorten your duration as outlined in chapter 8.

The aerobic exercise program just listed has as its primary goal to burn body fat through a six-days-per-week, low-intensity, long-duration program. I recommend that the program be walking since it is the most convenient, most practical, and easiest to monitor your heart rate. If you can't get all your walking in at one time each day, you can walk twice a day, perhaps thirty minutes in the morning and forty-five minutes at night. That is perfectly acceptable. If you desire, you could cut one day short by fifteen to thirty minutes and add fifteen to thirty minutes to another day. Saturday is often a good day to go for that extra long walk.

TABLE 15.2
Summary of Caloric Expenditure of Selected Physical Activities
(Calories Expended Per 30 Minutes)

ACTIVITY	BODY WEIGHT			
	100	140	180	220
Basketball (full court)	160	220	280	340
Bicycling (5.5 mph)	100	135	175	210
Bicycling (13 mph)	200	280	370	460
Golf (walking)	80	100	130	160
Racquetball (singles)	150	200	250	300
Walking (15 min/mile)	150	200	250	300
Jogging (10 min/mile)	240	320	400	480
Running (6 min/mile)	360	480	600	720
Swimming, crawl (50 yds/min)	200	270	340	410

The aerobic program will also begin to develop your cardiorespiratory fitness. This will progress slowly at first since the intensity is below 65 percent. But you are building a foundation for more rapid cardiorespiratory fitness gains later when you lose the fat and increase the intensity to 65 percent to 75 percent.

The Muscle-development Exercise Program

To complement the aerobic program, a muscle-development exercise program is an *absolute must*. Remember, the muscles burn the fat—the more muscles, the more fat that can be burned. Although the aerobics program will increase the ability of the muscle to burn more fat, that program alone will not develop muscles over the entire body. You will need to do light weight training and/or calisthenics on a regular basis to develop total body muscles.

Overfat persons do not need to modify the muscle-development program outlined in chapters 10 and 11. They can follow the weight-training program, the calisthenics program, or a combination of both. The only requirement is to faithfully start a regular two-day-per-week program and not neglect it. Weight training develops the muscles so that during the aerobics program they can burn the fat.

Weight-loss Quackery

Most persons want to look good, and they realize that excess fat is unhealthy. In their search for the "easy way" to lose weight, they try all kinds of products and methods that promise quick results. Quackery in the weight-loss business is extensive.

Spot Reduction

Spot reduction holds that if you have fat in a specific area of the body and if you exercise that spot, you will lose fat at that spot. Unfortunately, our bodies don't work that way. If you want to lose excess fat on the abdomen, you can do situps all day and you won't lose the fat. Situps will develop the muscles under the fat, but the fat will stay on top of the muscle. You cannot choose the location of the fat you want to lose from the body. To lose the fat over the muscle, you must do aerobic exercises such as walking. The walking will demand large amounts of energy, and the body will draw on the fat from wherever the greater amounts are deposited. So, walk to burn the fat on the abdomen, and do situps to develop the muscle under the fat.

Body Wrap, Saunas, and Sweat Suits

All three of these body-weight reduction aids have one thing in common: they elevate body temperature and cause you to lose body water, which will make it appear as though you lost weight. The weight is water and will be replaced when you drink fluids. These products can be dangerous for persons with heart trouble.

Protein Diets, Citrus Fruit Diets, and Caffeine

These also have one thing in common: they help you lose body water, which will appear as though you lost fat. When you go off the diet (high protein or citrus fruit), you will regain the water. Additionally, caffeine in coffee, tea, colas, soft drinks, and diet pills acts as a diuretic and increases water loss through the kidneys.

Rollers, Vibrating Belt

You cannot mechanically squeeze fat off your body. Fat can be eliminated only as you burn it off chemically through aerobic exercise. The rollers and vibrating belts may feel good and help reduce tension, but they won't get rid of any fat.

Special Foods

I am not aware of any scientific literature that supports any magical foods to help you lose body fat. Once again, you may lose water but not body fat. I am also not aware of any biochemical reason why foods can't be eaten together. The body can handle fats, carbohydrates, and proteins all eaten at the same time. It can also handle fruits mixed together.

Summary

The essential ingredient to help you lose fat is an aerobic and muscle-development exercise program. Gimmicks, fad diets, and pills may temporarily help you lose weight (usually water), but they won't solve the basic problem of excess fat and too little muscle. The body chemistry can be changed only through a sound exercise program. Don't expect quick changes. To change the body chemistry, to add muscle, to burn fat more efficiently, and to lose body fat will take months. If your body fat exceeds 30 percent for men and 40 percent for women, it may take more than a year to appreciably change your body chemistry. So, have patience.

Many students at ORU who are on our special walking program succeed in losing the necessary fat if they have patience, don't give up, and don't cut corners. Usually, before there is much weight loss, body fat and inches are lost. Bill was five feet nine inches, 235 pounds, and 34 percent fat. In his first fifteen weeks on the program he lost only four pounds. But he dropped 5 percent fat, two inches on his waist, and three inches on his hips. During the next fifteen weeks, the weight started coming off. He lost 3 percent fat and eighteen pounds. He had to develop muscle before he could really begin to see the weight come off.

Use the graph at the end of this chapter. Weigh yourself weekly and plot it. Don't be discouraged if you don't lose at first. Look at the overall trend.

Now that we have set the priority on the exercise program for effective fat control, let's look at diet. What we eat is also important.

Steps You Could Take (If you have excess body fat to lose)

1. What is your predicted maximum heart rate (see chap. 8)?
   _____

2. What is your heart rate at 55 percent and 65 percent of your maximum? 55% _____ , 65% _____

3. Refer to Table 15.1 in this chapter, and outline your aerobics exercise program to lose body fat over the next twenty-five weeks using the chart in chapter 8. Exercise six days per week.

4. Record your aerobic activity on the chart in chapter 8.

5. Describe the muscle-development program you will follow (refer to chaps. 10 and 11).

6. Record your weight changes each week on the graph below. Weigh yourself the same time of day and same day each week.

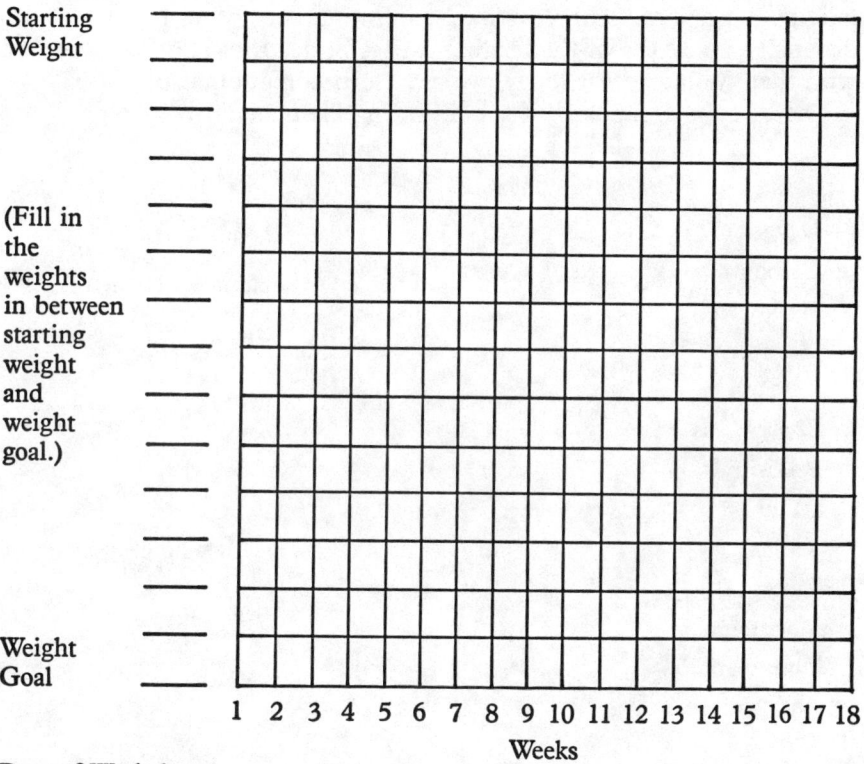

Starting Weight ____

(Fill in the weights in between starting weight and weight goal.)

Weight Goal ____

1 2 3 4 5 6 7 8 9 10 11 12 13 14 15 16 17 18
Weeks

Date of Week 1 _____

16

Basic Nutrients Needed for Health

Our health depends largely upon what we eat. Poor eating habits have been associated with hyperactivity of children, physical fatigue, mental fatigue, depression, stunted growth, and numerous other problems. Additionally, six to ten of the leading causes of death have been associated with diet. What we eat today, we tend to become tomorrow.

The body is composed of the following elements:

Element	Percent	
Element	*Percent*	
Oxygen	65	
Carbon	18	96% (Nonmetallic elements)
Hydrogen	10	
Nitrogen	3	
Calcium	1	
Phosphorus	1	
Potassium		
Sulfur		
Sodium	1	4% (Metallic elements)
Chlorine		
Magnesium		
More than 15 other elements	1	
	100	

These elements are constantly being depleted to provide energy for the body, to build new cells, to repair old cells, and to regulate the various body processes. Since we are unable to absorb these elements into our bodies through our skin, we must get them through food we eat and liquids we drink.

Nutrients

Nutrients are chemical parts of food and liquids that have specific functions in the body. The two overall functions of nutrients are (1) to provide essential elements the body needs to sustain life and (2) to provide energy for the body. The essential elements we need for health are found in six basic nutrients: carbohydrates, fats, proteins, vitamins, minerals, and water. Each nutrient will be discussed in detail later in this chapter.

Carbohydates, fats, and *proteins* are considered the main nutrients since you can receive all the essential vitamins and minerals with a proper balance of foods containing these three. Carbohydrates and fats are composed of carbon, oxygen, and hydrogen. Proteins are composed of those three elements plus nitrogen.

The energy we receive from the food we eat depends upon the amount of carbohydrates, fats, and proteins in the food. The amount of calories per gram of nutrient is shown in the following table.

TABLE 16.1
Energy Content of Nutrients

NUTRIENT	CALORIES PER GRAM
Carbohydrates	4
Proteins	4
Fats	9

Fats have more than twice the caloric content of carbohydrates and proteins. Therefore, if we have a diet high in fat, we will be consuming a lot of calories. Some diets purported to cause weight loss restrict carbohydrates. As can be seen, carbohydrates are not the problem. In an earlier chapter we gave the comparison of skim milk having 65 fewer calories per cup than whole milk. Skim milk has all the nutrients of whole milk except the fat. A 6.5-ounce can of tuna packed in oil is 433 calories, but the same tuna packed in water contains only 200 calories. Both have the exact same amount of protein. Reducing your fat intake can greatly reduce your caloric intake.

Functions of Carbohydrates, Fats, and Proteins

The primary function of *carbohydrates* is to provide all the cells of the body with *energy*. While most cells use a combination of both fats and carbohydrates for energy, brain and nerve tissue use *only* carbohydrates for energy. Muscle cells use a combination of carbohydrates and fats for energy. However, if your cells are working at a high energy demand as in jogging fast, sprinting, or swimming under water, only carbohydrates are used for energy since fat metabolism requires more oxygen. Often at high levels of exercise not enough oxygen is consumed to metabolize fat.

Carbohydrates must be present in the diet in order for fats to be used for energy. If a person is on a diet that restricts carbohydrates and the body is deprived of them, proteins will be converted into carbohydrates to meet this need. Because this tears down muscle tissue and is not beneficial to our bodies, we must get the necessary carbohydrates in our diets to prevent our body proteins from being converted into the needed carbohydrates. On the other hand, excess carbohydrates in the diet are converted to fat and stored.

Fats provide the cells of the body, except brain and nerve cells, with energy. At rest about two-thirds of the cells' energy come from fat and one-third from carbohydrates. Excess fat in the diet is stored in fat cells. Some storage of fat in the body is important for reserve energy (5 percent to 15 percent for men, 15 percent to 25 percent for women).

Fats are also important as a carrier of vitamins A, D, E, and K, a protector of vital body organs, and an insulator of the body. They are also an important part of cell walls and hormones, and they serve to depress appetite.

The major function of *proteins* is to build, repair, and maintain cells. They form the major part of muscle tissue and are essential for muscle contraction. They are an important part of hemoglobin as well as numerous hormones. Excess proteins in the diet are converted to fat and stored. In emergencies, proteins can be converted to carbohydrates and used for energy. Our daily need of protein is about one gram per kilogram of body weight for the normal adult and two grams per kilogram of body weight for the adolescent and body builder.

Intake of Carbohydrates, Fats, and Proteins

To meet the body requirements, all three nutrients must be included in the daily diet. The ratio of the three main nutrients in the diet is very important. Americans are currently eating too much fat and the wrong kind of carbohydrates. Changes need to be made in our diet to improve our health. Our protein intake needs to stay about the same, our fat intake needs to decrease, and our carbohydrate intake needs to increase. In terms of calories, it is obvious that we need to reduce our fat intake.

TABLE 16.2
Dietary Intake of
Carbohydrates, Fats, and Proteins

CURRENT DIET	PERCENT	RECOMMENDED DIET	PERCENT
Carbohydrates	45	Carbohydrates	70
Starch	22	Starch	55
Sugar	23	Sugar	15
Fats	40	Fats	15
Saturated	25	Saturated	3
Unsaturated	15	Unsaturated	12
Proteins	15	Proteins	15
	100		100

Carbohydrates: Simple Versus Complex

Carbohydrates are basically of two types: simple and complex. Simple carbohydrates consist of sugars, and complex carbohydrates consist of starch and cellulose (fiber). Actually, a complex carbohydrate is many sugars combined together.

Sugars are of six common types: (1) sucrose—table sugar, found in sugar beets and sugar cane; (2) fructose—sugar found in fruits and honey; (3-4) galactose and lactose—sugar found in milk; (5) maltose—sugar found in grains and cereals; and (6) glucose—sugar found in fruits, corn syrup, and honey.

Food manufacturers are required to list the ingredients of each product on its label. Sometimes rather than one of these six names, another term will be used, such as brown sugar, honey, corn syrup, levulose, or dextrose. Regardless of the name, they are sugars, and the body handles them as sugars. Some persons have attempted to lower their sugar intake by switching to honey. Unfortunately, honey has more calories than regular sugar. One tablespoon of honey has sixty-two calories, and one tablespoon of sugar has forty-eight.

Starch is made up of many sugars chemically combined. As many as three hundred sugars may be combined to make a starch. Starch is primarily found in vegetables, grains, seeds, and fruits.

The current American diet is too low in total carbohydrates but too high in sugar. Each year Americans have been eating more sugar. Nowhere is this more obvious than in the soft drink industry, as illustrated by the following table.

TABLE 16.3
Soft Drink Consumption
from 1935 to 1980

YEAR	12 OUNCE CANS OR BOTTLES CONSUMED PER PERSON PER YEAR
1935	40
1965	145
1980	300

Of the carbohydrates we eat, approximately 50 percent come from starches, 40 percent from sucrose (table sugar), 5 percent from galactose and lactose (milk sugar), and 5 percent from glucose, maltose, and fructose (vegetables and fruits). The amount of carbohydrates we receive from starch should be increased from 50 percent to 75 percent, the sugar we get from vegetables and fruits should be increased from 5 percent to 10 percent, milk sugar can stay the same at 5 percent, and the sugar from table sugar should be reduced from 40 percent to 10 percent. Why should we reduce our sugar and increase our starch intake?

The Sugar Problem

Excess sugar in the diet causes several problems. This can be seen by reviewing how the body digests carbohydrates (see Fig. 16.1).

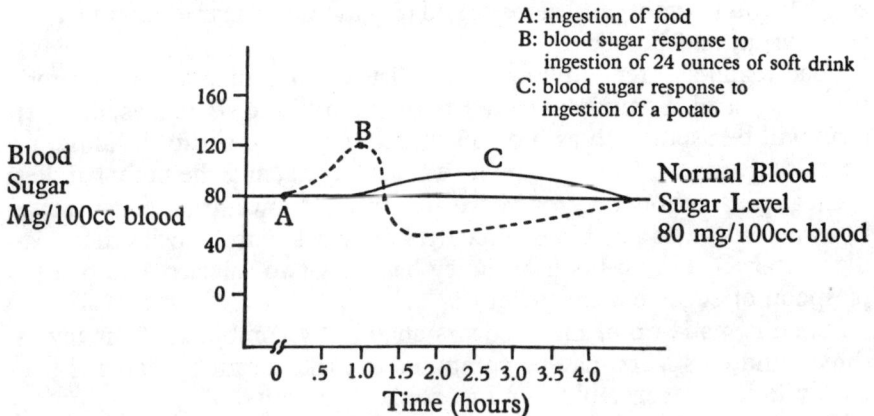

A: ingestion of food
B: blood sugar response to ingestion of 24 ounces of soft drink
C: blood sugar response to ingestion of a potato

Normal Blood Sugar Level 80 mg/100cc blood

Blood Sugar Mg/100cc blood

Time (hours)

Fig. 16.1. Blood Sugar Response to Ingestion of Sugar and of Complex Carbohydrate

Complex carbohydrates in the form of starch are not directly absorbed into the blood; only simple sugars are. Therefore, when carbohydrates are eaten, enzymes in the mouth, stomach, and small intestine begin to break the carbohydrates down into their simplest form—sugar. When this has been accomplished, in the small intestine the sugar can pass through the intestinal wall, be absorbed by the blood stream, and be carried to the cells of the body. To break a starch down into its simplest form takes time. Since starches take longer to be digested than a simple sugar, they pass more slowly into the blood stream, and the body can easily handle the slow flow of sugar being absorbed.

On the other hand, when a sugar is eaten, first, it passes very rapidly through the digestive tract to the blood stream and causes a sudden increase in blood sugar. The body is extremely sensitive to blood sugar increases or decreases. This rapid increase stimulates a release of insulin from the pancreas, and because it is reacting to the rapid blood sugar increase, the insulin is often released in excess of need. Insulin's function is to transport the sugar out of the blood into the cells of the body. If the cells don't need all the sugar immediately for energy, the sugar is changed into fat and stored. Therefore, high-sugar diets can lead to increased body fat.

Second, the excess insulin released causes the liver to produce triglycerides and very low-density lipoproteins and release them into the blood. This can accelerate atherosclerosis. Hence, excess sugar can lead to cardiovascular problems, especially hardening of the arteries.

Third, the excess insulin will do its job too well and transport so much sugar out of the blood and into the cells that the blood sugar will reverse itself and rapidly drop below normal (hypoglycemia). This low blood sugar causes weakness and stimulates hunger. The person then tends to eat when it is really not necessary. Therefore, a high-sugar diet leads to a craving for more sugar.

Fourth, over a period of years, the up-and-down effect of high blood sugar and high insulin levels followed by low blood sugar and low insulin can cause the cell to reject the insulin that is carrying the sugar into the cell. In time the blood sugar is elevated and stays high, and a condition of diabetes develops. The cell actually has become insensitive to the insulin. Most adult-onset diabetes is due to this factor and is caused by the person's dietary habits.

Fifth, when your diet contains excess sugar, especially table sugar that is added to soft drinks, bakery goods, and similar products, you are robbing your cells of important nutrients. Table sugar is empty calories; that is, it contains the calories necessary to provide the body with energy, but it contains no vitamins or minerals. When you receive your carbohydrates through starches, you also receive the vitamins and minerals in those foods. Even when your carbohydrates come from sugar in fruits and milk, you at least get some vitamins and minerals. You may receive all the calories you need to live, but an excessive sugar intake may cause you to be overweight *and* malnourished. You may also suffer the disease of malnutrition.

Low-carbohydrate Diets

Low-carbohydrate diets that some persons advocate for weight loss are not only contrary to the needs of the body for good health but are also inconsistent with the Scriptures. When Adam was created upon the earth, God gave him a diet of fruits, vegetables, and grains—a high-carbohydrate diet. God said, "See, I have given you every herb that yields seed which is on the face of all the earth, and every tree whose fruit yields seed; to you it shall be for food" (Gen. 1:29).

Our bodies were made to function on a high-carbohydrate, high-starch diet with the starch coming from vegetables, fruits, and grains. A diet high in these elements provides not only all the carbohydrates you need but also vitamins, minerals, and most of the necessary protein and fat.

Carbohydrates are an absolute must in the diet because the brain and nerve tissue can use only carbohydrates as fuel for energy. Low-carbohydrate diets can lead to mental fatigue and slow reflexes because of low blood sugar.

Loss of body salt and body water is also a result of a low-carbohydrate diet. This can lead to body dehydration and weakness. The weight loss from this diet is often not fat but water. When the diet is stopped, the water will again be retained by the body and weight will be regained.

If the body is short of needed nutrients, it has an amazing ability to convert other nutrients into what is needed. A low-carbohydrate diet lowers blood sugar. Since body balance requires an adequate amount of blood sugar, the liver will convert protein into the needed sugar. Therefore, on a low-carbohydrate diet, the weight you lose may be not only water, but also a loss of protein in the muscle tissue. This is detrimental to optimal health because the protein is needed to build and maintain vital body structures.

Usually a low-carbohydrate diet means other foods must be eaten to replace the carbohydrates. Unfortunately, this means an increase in fat and protein intake, which can lead to serious health problems as will be discussed later.

Steps You Could Take

Foods that are good carbohydrate sources are those high in starch and low in sugar. The average American eats more than one hundred pounds of table sugar per year, and that must be reduced to have good health. The following foods should be emphasized or de-emphasized to accomplish this objective.

Emphasize Starch	*De-emphasize Sugar*
Fresh fruits	Table sugar
Fresh vegetables	Candy
Seeds (sunflower, sesame,	Soft drinks
flax, etc.)	Presweetened cereals
Grains	Bakery goods (cakes, pies,
Nuts	doughnuts, cookies)
Unsweetened cereals	
Bread (whole grain or multigrain)	
Baked potatoes and brown rice	

Fiber

Fiber is a type of complex carbohydrate of which cellulose is the most common. Fiber, also called roughage or bulk, is found primarily in fruits, vegetables, and grains. Since the body does not possess the enzymes necessary to break down fiber, it is not digested by the body. It passes through the small and large intestine relatively unchanged and is eliminated in bowel movements.

Years ago when scientists began to evaluate foods, they discovered that the fiber in foods, especially grains, was not being digested by the body. Since it was not digested, they concluded erroneously that fiber had no value in the diet, and they began to eliminate it from foods. Wheat, which is the most important grain in the world and widely used in cereals and breads, was refined. The fiber from it was eliminated. Over the past ten to twenty years the folly of that decision has been realized.

Function of Fiber

Although several specific purposes of fiber have been established, much is yet to be learned about its importance in the diet. We do know that it promotes regular bowel movements. Fiber absorbs water in the large intestine, and the stools are softer and larger. They leave the body easily with no need of straining or pushing. Constipation is rare among people with high-fiber diets. The straining caused by hard stools can lead to hemorrhoids and possible hernias.

High-fiber diets also quicken the transit time of food from intake to elimination. Transit time of food in persons on a high-fiber diet is approximately one-third that of persons with low-fiber diets. Authorities recommend two bowel movements a day. Waste products of metabolism stay in the large intestine three times longer with a low-fiber diet. This allows the waste products, some of which are toxic chemicals and may be carcinogenic (cancer causing), a longer time to irritate the large intestine. This may be a strong factor in diverticular disease, colitis, and colon cancer.

Lack of fiber in the diet has also been associated with high cholesterol, appendicitis, gallbladder diseases, diabetes, and obesity. Fiber is an absolutely essential part of a healthful diet, not so much for what it causes but for what it prevents. As reported in an earlier chapter, Seventh-Day Adventists have much less cancer than the general population. This may be partially attributed to their emphasis on a vegetarian diet with a good supply of fiber.

Sources of Fiber

The amount of fiber needed daily in the diet has not been established. A typical American eats four to eight grams daily, but vegetarians eat as much as twenty to thirty grams. Perhaps a safe amount is at least twenty to twenty-five grams per day. If a person does not normally have two bowel movements per day with the stool soft, chances are there is not enough fiber in the diet.

The sources of fiber should vary. Bran found in grains serves as one of the best sources of fiber. However, if the grain has been refined, the bran is lost and the fiber is gone. After a food is refined, some of the vitamins and minerals are restored (enriched) and occasionally additional vitamins are added (fortified), but the fiber is still absent. Therefore, unrefined grains are best in order to receive the fiber they possess.

While bran from grains is a good fiber source, at least half the fiber should come from vegetables and fruits. Cooked vegetables and fruits, however, lose some of their fiber. Therefore, we should eat vegetables and fruits raw if possible.

Since breakfast cereals are an excellent source of fiber *if properly selected,* the following table lists the breakdown of carbohydrates in selected high-fiber cereals.

TABLE 16.4
Selected High-fiber Breakfast Cereals

CEREAL (1 SERVING)	TOTAL CARBOHYDRATES (GRAMS)	STARCH (GRAMS)	SUGAR (GRAMS)	FIBER (GRAMS)
All Bran	21	7	5	9
Corn Bran	24	13	6	5
Bran Chex	29	13	11	5
40% Bran Flakes	23	14	5	4
Raisin Bran	28	12	12	4
Most	22	12	6	4
Cracklin' Bran	20	8	8	4
Total	23	18	3	2
Wheaties	23	18	3	2
Nutrigrain	24	20	2	2
Wheat Chex	23	19	2	2
Quaker Oats	20	18	0	2
Shredded Wheat	24	22	0	2
Cheerios	20	19	1	2

I emphasize the need to select a breakfast cereal with as much fiber and as little sugar as possible. The next table lists many other cereals and the amounts of starch, sugar, and fiber.

TABLE 16.5
Other Breakfast Cereals

CEREAL (1 SERVING)	TOTAL CARBOHYDRATES (GRAMS)	STARCH (GRAMS)	SUGAR (GRAMS)	FIBER (GRAMS)
Kix	24	22	2	0
Special K	21	19	2	0
Rice Chex	25	23	2	0
Corn Flakes	25	23	2	0
Rice Krispies	25	22	3	0
Product 19	24	21	3	0
Grape Nuts	23	20	3	0
Life	19.4	13	6	.4
Wheat & Raisins	23.4	13	10	.4
Cocoa Puffs	25	14	11	0
Frosted Flakes	26	15	11	0
Honey Comb	25	14	11	0
Trix	25	13	12	0

CEREAL (1 SERVING)	TOTAL CARBOHYDRATES (GRAMS)	STARCH (GRAMS)	SUGAR (GRAMS)	FIBER (GRAMS)
Sugar Corn Pops	26	14	12	0
Fruit Loops	25	12	13	0
Apple Jacks	26	12	14	0
Sugar Crisp	26	12	14	0

How you choose your breakfast can influence your health. A breakfast of Corn Bran, Bran Chex, or 40% Bran Flakes topped with strawberries or a banana and no sugar added can start you off with low sugar, high starch, and high fiber. On the other hand, a breakfast with a sugar-coated cereal starts you off with high sugar, low starch, and no fiber.

TABLE 16.6
Fiber in Selected Fruits, Vegetables, and Grains

FOOD	FIBER (GRAMS)
Raspberries, red, ¾ cup	3
Broccoli, 1 medium stalk	6
Apple, 1 medium	5
Spinach, ½ cup	5
Banana, 1 medium	2
Orange, 1 medium	2
Strawberries, ½ cup	1
Cabbage, ½ cup	4
Prunes, 6 medium	2
Peas, ½ cup	3
Potato, 1 medium	3
Lima beans, ¼ cup	2
Kidney beans, ½ cup	3
String beans, ⅔ cup	1
Carrots, ¾ cup	1
Beets, ½ cup	1
Whole (100%) wheat bread, 2 slices	2
White enriched bread, 2 slices	.2
Almonds, ¼ cup	5

Fiber may be fabulous, but too much of any good thing can lead to problems. Excess fiber in the diet can lead to diarrhea and cause dehydration and mineral loss.

Steps You Could Take

1. Eat high fiber cereals topped with fresh fruit for breakfast every day.

2. Have at least two raw fruits every day, preferably one an apple.

3. Have spinach, broccoli, or cabbage in a salad as many days as possible.

4. Analyze your diet. You should attempt to eat twenty to twenty-five grams of fiber per day.

Fats

Excess fat in the diet spells double trouble. But notice, I said excess. Some fat in the diet is essential for life. The problem that we face, however, is too much fat in our diets. At the turn of the century, fat accounted for 25 percent to 30 percent of Americans' daily caloric intake compared to 40 percent to 45 percent today. Teen-agers, who tend to have poor dietary habits, often have 50 percent fat in their diets. The double trouble that excess fat intake causes is (1) excess body fat and obesity (fat has more than double the calories of an equal amount of carbohydrates or proteins) and (2) elevated blood fats. We have previously asserted that the chief cause of heart attack and stroke is atherosclerosis. A major contributing factor to atherosclerosis is high blood fats. We need to reduce our fat intake, but we also need to be aware of the types of fats in foods. Some fats appear to cause more health problems than others. The Scriptures teach us, "This shall be a perpetual statute throughout your generations in all your dwellings: you shall eat neither fat nor blood" (Lev. 3:17).

Types of Fats

Triglycerides are the most common fats we eat. These are of two basic types: saturated and unsaturated. *Saturated* triglycerides, or saturated fats, are found primarily in animal products. Meat products, such as beef, pork, lamb, lobster, and shrimp, dairy products, such as milk, cheese, butter, and cream, and eggs have high quantities of saturated fat. Although fats are essential for health, saturated fats are not and should be reduced in the diet.

Unsaturated fats, some of which are polyunsaturated, do not appear to cause health problems to the same degree that saturated fats do. They are found primarily in vegetables. Safflower, corn, peanuts, soybeans, and cotton seed are often made into oils used in baking, in cooking, and in making margarine. They are all high in unsaturated fats. Coconut oil, however, is more highly saturated and should be avoided or de-emphasized in the diet.

Another type of fat is *cholesterol,* which is needed for body functioning. In fact, the liver manufactures some cholesterol. It is found in almost all cells and is a basic structure for several hormones. It is normally present in the blood. Recently, cholesterol has been further analyzed in terms of its component parts. When cholesterol is measured in the blood, it can be measured as a total quantity, or it can be analyzed as high-density cholesterol (HDL) and low-density cholesterol (LDL). The type of cholesterol your blood carries is perhaps equally important as is the total cholesterol. Studies have shown that LDL is harmful and HDL may actually be beneficial. The good news is that aerobic exercise programs of sufficient duration increase HDL levels and decrease LDL. To be effective, however, the aerobic program needs to be followed at least five days per week for a minimum of thirty to forty-five minutes each day for possibly six months or longer.

Blood Fats and Atherosclerosis

The preponderance of evidence supports the findings that the higher the blood fats, the greater the atherosclerosis. Having high blood fats, triglycerides, and cholesterol appears to be related to several factors.

1. *Body fat.* The greater the body fat, the greater the blood fats. Therefore, you should avoid excess body fat as was described earlier.

2. *Diet.* Diets high in saturated fats and cholesterol seem to contribute to elevated blood fats. Therefore, reduce your intake of these substances.

3. *Heredity.* Certain persons have genetic weaknesses that prevent their properly handling blood fats. Occasionally a person has no excess body fat, has a good diet, and exercises but still has high blood fats. In all probability that person has a genetic weakness. If that is your problem, you may need a physician's assistance.

4. *Inactivity.* Persons who are physically inactive and who don't exercise tend to have higher blood-fat levels than persons who are active and who regularly do aerobic exercises.

5. *Stress.* Stress tends to elevate blood fats. Tax consultants have been found to have elevated blood-fats around April 15 when they are under high pressure to get tax returns completed.

The amount of triglycerides and cholesterol permitted in the blood before atherosclerosis begins to develop cannot be absolutely predicted. The following table indicates acceptable blood-fat ranges. Have your physician evaluate your blood fat. If you are in the very poor category, all indications are that you are a prime candidate for the development of atherosclerosis. Exercise, watch your fat intake, and lose body fat. Check with your physician and ask what else you can do.

TABLE 16.7
Acceptable Blood-fat Levels

HEALTH FITNESS STANDARD	MILLIGRAMS/100 CUBIC CENTIMETERS OF BLOOD		RATIO OF TOTAL CHOLESTEROL TO HDL
	TRIGLYCERIDES	CHOLESTEROL	
Excellent	20–40	100–150	3.0
Good	40–60	150–200	4.0
Acceptable	60–100	200–240	5.0
Poor	100–150	240–280	6.0
Very poor	150–plus	280–plus	7.0–plus

Dietary Fat Sources

You should reduce your overall intake of fat by emphasizing certain foods and de-emphasizing or avoiding others. By substituting low-fat meat and milk products, you can significantly reduce your fat intake. A small difference in potato selection will make a tremendous difference in fat intake. One baked potato is 100 calories, but one cup of French fries is 480 calories. One cup of whole milk is 150 calories compared to 85 calories in one cup of skim milk. The difference in calories is exclusively due to the fat in the fried potatoes and the whole milk. Chocolate is 75 percent fat and should be de-emphasized.

Steps You Could Take

1. Have your blood cholesterol and triglycerides evaluated by your physician. Cholesterol _____ , Triglycerides _____ , Total Cholesterol/HDL Ratio _____

2. What is the health fitness standard of each?

3. Limit your fat intake to 15 percent of your total daily caloric intake. This would mean approximately fifteen to twenty grams for a person on a thousand calorie per day intake to fifty to sixty grams for a person on a three thousand calorie per day intake. Read the labels of foods you eat to determine your daily fat intake in grams.

4. If you eat foods high in starch, such as vegetables, fruits, and grains, you will also get the fat you need and it will be in the unsaturated form. Medical science is discovering the truth in what the Scriptures said centuries ago. God clearly declared that we should not eat fat

(see Lev. 3:17) and He approved certain meat products but forbade others (see Lev. 11:3–12). Several of the meats that He stated we should not eat have been discovered to be high in fat, especially pork and shellfish (shrimp, crab, lobster). Many people feel they need meat for protein. You can get all the protein you need by eating only the low-fat foods listed below.

Low-fat Foods to Emphasize	High-fat Foods to De-emphasize
Ice milk	Cream
Sherbets	Ice cream
Skim milk	Whole milk
Fish	Egg yolks
Chicken and turkey	Beef
(without the skin)	Pork
Low-calorie salad dressings	Lamb
Weight Watchers' products	Shellfish
	Fried foods
	Butter and margarine
	Regular salad dressings

Protein

The average American eats too much meat. We have come to believe we need a good supply of meat in order to get the amount of protein we need. Most people plan their meals around the meat they are serving. At a restaurant, the main entree is usually meat. Actually, our daily need is one gram of protein per kilogram of body weight. That means adults need only three to four ounces of protein per day to meet all their protein needs.

The Problem with a High-protein Diet

Several potential health problems are associated with a high-protein diet. Persons on a high-protein diet eat an excess amount of meat. The high-meat diet will result not only in excess protein consumption but also in high fat intake, with the fat being in the form of cholesterol and saturated fat which is found in meat. We have already described the double trouble of a high-fat diet. Beef is 20 percent to 40 percent fat. Pork has similar percentages of fat. Chicken and turkey without the skins are the best meat for protein, since they contain only 10 percent to 15 percent fat.

The excess protein in the diet does not build excess cells. Rather, the protein not needed for cell repair is converted in the liver to fat and stored in fat cells.

When the body converts protein to fat, ammonia is produced. Since ammonia is toxic to the body, it is changed into urea and eliminated by the kidney in the urine. Since urea is also toxic, water is drawn from the body cells to dilute it, and excess water is lost from the body in the urine.

Therefore, a high-protein diet can cause the body to lose excess amounts of body water, leading to dehydration. Many persons on high-protein diets enjoy quick and large weight losses. However, they are being fooled! The weight loss is only water, not fat, and will return as soon as the diet is ended.

Not only do high-protein diets produce a false sense of weight loss, but they can precipitate serious health problems because you are not getting the vitamins and minerals you need and you may become dehydrated. It has been reported that at least sixty deaths have been directly related to high-protein diets used by persons to lose weight.

Your body is the temple of God! It was made in a precise way, and it needs a balance of carbohydrates, fats, and proteins. When any of the three is deficient or in excess, health problems may develop.

Did God Create Man a Vegetarian?

In Genesis 1:29 we read, "See, I have given you every herb that yields seed which is on the face of all the earth, and every tree whose fruit yields seed; to you it shall be for food." Many people believe God's original intent was for man to be a vegetarian, that is, to eat only vegetables, fruits, and grains, not meat. As time went by, God limited man's days to 120 years (see Gen. 6:3) and added meat to man's diet (see Gen. 9:3). The levitical laws further spelled out the limits of acceptable and unacceptable meats.

The basic units, or building blocks, of proteins are amino acids. There are twenty-three different amino acids that can be combined in numerous ways to make a single protein. Ten amino acids cannot be synthesized by the body and are called "essential" amino acids. A complete protein is one that contains all the essential amino acids, whereas an incomplete protein does not contain all the essential amino acids.

We can get all the essential amino acids we need without eating meat. Daniel demonstrated that with only vegetables and water he could fare better than the others on the king's meat (see Dan. 1:8–19). A very important point, however, is that the vegetarian must emphasize a *variety* of foods in the diet, especially soybeans, peas, lentils, and beans, and must supplement these with cheese, milk, and eggs. When a variety of nonmeat foods are eaten, all the protein necessary can be attained. The only nutrient missing in a vegetarian diet is vitamin B_{12}. This can be obtained through a vitamin supplement.

Steps You Could Take

1. The following foods should be emphasized or de-emphasized as a source of protein:

Protein Sources to Emphasize	Protein Sources to De-emphasize
Chicken and turkey, without skin, baked	Pork, lamb
	Organ meat, such as liver
Tuna fish packed in water	Beef
Fish, baked	Shellfish
Skim milk	Whole milk
Low-fat cheeses	Egg yolks
Peanuts, almonds, walnuts*	
Beans, peas, lentils, soybeans	
Egg whites	

*Limit the nut intake because of their fat content.

2. The table below lists common vegetable protein sources. To have a meal with all the essential amino acids, when you choose an item from Row 1, choose another item for the same meal in Row 2 of the same column.

1	Legumes and	Rice and	Noodles and	Wheat and
2	Dairy products Grains Seeds Nuts Corn	Dairy products Legumes Peas Nuts Wheat	Wheat Nuts Dairy products (e.g., macaroni and cheese)	Legumes Seeds Peanuts (e.g., peanut butter sand- wich) Dairy products (e.g., cereal and milk)

Vitamins and Minerals

Vitamins and minerals are basic for optimal health. Since the body cannot manufacture them, they must be ingested daily into the body. How much we need each day has been established by the National Research Council of the Food and Drug Administration. The daily need has been expressed as the *Recommended Daily Allowances* (RDA), and it is revised periodically as new research becomes available.

Although taking less than the RDA for an extended period of time may lead to a health problem, an excess of the RDA will not make you healthier. In fact, consistent excess of certain vitamins can lead to medical problems. Americans spend nearly $500 million each year on vitamin and mineral supplements, most of which exceed the body's needs.

I believe the excess use of vitamins today stems from man's basic nature to desire health and his attempt to achieve it in the easiest way possible. Some people take pills because they think that is the easy way to cure their health problems. The cure to most problems, however, is not a pill but a disciplined lifestyle of exercise, good nutrition, and other important behaviors.

In the United States health problems due to a vitamin deficiency are rare. It is amazing how many people do not exercise and do not control their intake of sugar, fat, and salt, all of which relate directly to heart disease—America's number one killer. Yet they pop numerous vitamin pills, which are not related to any current health problems.

Vitamins: Body Needs and Sources

Two major categories of vitamins are fat-soluble and water-soluble. *Fat-soluble vitamins* are A, D, E, and K, and they must be ingested with fat. If no fat is present, they will pass out of the digestive tract and will not be absorbed into the body. Therefore, when you take a vitamin supplement, it is best to take it with a meal. Once absorbed into the body, fat-soluble vitamins can be stored in fat, muscles, and the liver to be used when needed.

Water-soluble vitamins are readily absorbed into the body but are just as readily passed out of the body in urine and perspiration. They are not stored in the body and, therefore, need to be ingested daily. Water-soluble vitamins include B_1, B_2, B_6, B_{12}, C, niacin, pantothenic acid, biotin, and folacin.

Vitamins have a wide variety of functions in the body. They help regulate nearly all metabolic reactions, they help convert carbohydrates and fat into energy, and they assist with bone and tissue repairs. The following table summarizes each vitamin.

TABLE 16.8
Vitamin Summary

VITAMIN	ADULT RDA	PRIMARY BODY FUNCTION	MAJOR SOURCE
A	5000 IU[1]	Tissue growth and repair, especially skin and all membranes; night vision	Vegetables, especially carrots, sweet potatoes, spinach; cantaloupe, pumpkin, and watermelon

VITAMIN	ADULT RDA	PRIMARY BODY FUNCTION	MAJOR SOURCE
D	500 IU	Bone calcification	Fortified milk, fish; the "sunshine" vitamin since it is naturally formed in the body in reaction to the sun's rays
E	30IU	Functions as an antioxidant to prevent cell-membrame damage; *may* help to delay the aging process; *may* help to prevent scar tissue	Wheat germ, walnuts, safflower, sunflower, cottonseed, almonds
K	1000 IU	Necessary to assist in the clotting of blood to prevent excess bleeding after a cut	Vegetables, especially lettuce, spinach, cauliflower, and cabbage
B_1 Thiamine	1.4 mg^2	Important in carbohydrate metabolism, which gives us energy	Brewer's yeast, wheat germ, sunflower seeds, soybeans, rice, peanuts, pecans, sesame seeds
B_2 Riboflavin	1.6 mg	Important in the metabolism of nutrients to give us energy; needed for healthy skin	Brewer's yeast, wheat germ, liver, cheese, soybeans
B_3 Niacin	18 mg	Converts proteins and fats into energy when needed	Brewer's yeast, soybeans, sesame seed, fish, chicken, wheat germ, sunflower
B_5 Pantothenic Acid	10 mg	Important for obtaining energy from carbohydrates, fats, and proteins; helps in the transmission of nerve impulses	Brewer's yeast, liver, eggs, fish, milk, wheat germ, rice, peanuts, broccoli, sweet potatoes
B_6 Pyridoxine	2.0 mg	Break down and produce proteins	Brewer's yeast, wheat germ, sunflower seeds, liver, fish, soybeans, beans, rice
B_{12}	.003 mg	Essential for the formation of red blood cells	Liver, fish, meat, eggs, dairy products; not found in plant products

VITAMIN	ADULT RDA	PRIMARY BODY FUNCTION	MAJOR SOURCE
C Ascorbic Acid	60 mg	Holds body cells together; strengthens blood vessels; helps wounds to heal; *may* assist in fighting infections and viruses	Fruits and vegetables, especially oranges, strawberries, lemons, grapefruit, cantaloupe, turnip greens, broccoli, Brussels sprouts, cauliflower, spinach, and cabbage
Biotin	.05 mg	Necessary for fatty-acid production and metabolism of proteins	Liver, eggs, mushrooms, peanuts, Brewer's yeast, wheat germ, fish, soybeans
Folacin	.4 mg	Necessary for the production of essential body proteins such as hemoglobin, nucleoproteins (DNA, RNA)	Brewer's yeast, soybeans, peanuts, wheat germ, spinach, oranges, pinto beans

[1]IU   international unit
[2]mg   milligram

Minerals: Body Needs and Sources

Minerals comprise 4 percent of the body weight and are essential for many vital body processes. Not only are minerals needed for health, but the proper balance among minerals is critical. Minerals work closely together, and each affects the other. Mineral imbalances can cause dehydration, heart attacks, and many other health problems.

Minerals are divided into two categories: macrominerals and trace minerals. *Macrominerals* are those for which we have a large daily requirement, such as calcium, phosphorus, sodium, chlorine, potassium, magnesium, and sulfur. The specific role of the macrominerals in the body is fairly well understood. *Trace minerals* are needed daily in smaller amounts. These include copper, iodine, zinc, iron, manganese, and more than fifteen others. Less is known about these trace minerals.

The following table outlines the minerals and their RDA, primary body function, and major dietary source.

TABLE 16.9
Mineral Summary

MINERAL	ADULT RDA	PRIMARY BODY FUNCTION	MAJOR SOURCE
Calcium	800 mg[1]	Needed for bone and teeth formation, nerve transmission, and blood clotting	Milk, cheese, sesame seeds, salmon, broccoli
Phosphorus	800 mg	Needed for bone and teeth formation and to maintain the acid-base balance in the blood	Milk, cheese, fish, meat, nuts, eggs, whole wheat, beans
Sodium	2.5 gm[2]	Needed for nerve transmission; to maintain water balance and the acid-base balance in the blood	Common salt, processed foods
Chlorine	2.0 gm	To maintain the acid-base balance in the blood and to form stomach acid (hydrochloric acid)	Common salt, processed foods
Potassium	2.5 gm	Functions with sodium to maintain the acid-base balance and water balance; to transmit nerve impulses	Processed foods, abundant in most foods both animal and plants
Magnesium	350 gm	Part of enzymes that metabolizes nutrients into energy; helps regulate body temperature; involved in the synthesis of proteins	Wheat germ, soybeans, peanuts, walnuts, spinach
Sulfur	Not Stated	Important part of all proteins	Protein foods
Iron	10 mg	Important part of hemoglobin	Eggs, liver, whole grains, beans
Copper	2 mg	Helps to combine iron with hemoglobin	Fish, nuts, beans
Fluorine	2 mg	Helps prevent tooth decay	Fish, most drinking water

MINERAL	ADULT RDA	PRIMARY BODY FUNCTION	MAJOR SOURCE
Zinc	15 mg	Associated with insulin and involved in carbohydrate metabolism	Wheat germ, soybeans, nuts
Iodine	15 mg	Important part of thyroid hormones	Fish, dairy products, vegetables
Silicon			
Vanadium			
Tin			
Nickel			
Selenium		Needed daily in the diet in very small quantities. Fish, dairy products, vegetables, wheat germ, and grains are the best overall sources.	
Manganese			
Molybdenum			
Cobalt			
Chromium			

¹mg milligram
²gm gram

Should We Supplement?

If we could be assured that we were receiving all the nutrients we needed through our diets, we would not need to supplement. Some persons may receive all they need, but most probably do not. When many foods are cooked, refined, or peeled, they lose important vitamins and minerals. Food we eat today may be grown in mineral-deficient soil. Therefore, even if we eat raw fruits or vegetables with the skin, we may be missing some of the vitamins and minerals found in those foods grown in good soil.

I recommend taking one multivitamin plus mineral supplement per day. The pill should include all the vitamins and minerals discussed here. Despite numerous testimonials and claims that large doses of vitamins can cure and prevent a variety of problems from the common cold to cancer and heart disease, the abundance of scientific research does not support those claims. One multivitamin plus mineral supplement per day with 100 percent RDA, or at most 200 percent RDA, is a good insurance policy against any possible deficiency and will not cause an overdose.

Consistent large doses (megavitamin usage tenfold over the RDA) can lead to overdose health problems. Kidney stones can result from excess vitamin C. Another potential problem is in the fat-soluble vitamins (A, E, D, K), which are stored in the body and can build up with continued overdoses.

Three exceptions to this one-a-day recommendation *may* include, first, the use of vitamin C. If you feel a cold developing, two hundred fifty to five hundred milligrams of vitamin C *may* help your body fight off the cold. This quantity is not a large dose. Second, women past age forty should take extra calcium—a calcium supplement of calcium carbonate (five hundred to one thousand milligrams). And the final exceptions are special situations, such as prolonged illness, pregnancy, lactation, or a high-level training program. Perhaps double the RDA is appropriate in these situations. Check with a physician to make sure.

Although one multivitamin plus mineral supplement per day may ensure that you receive all the vitamins and minerals you need each day, nothing replaces a good balanced diet of fresh fruits, vegetables, whole grains, and low-fat protein products. Also, there is no caloric value in vitamin pills. Persons who pop vitamin pills in the morning for extra energy rather than having a well-balanced breakfast are doing their body more harm than good.

Is Natural Better?

Sorry, but it appears that the body doesn't know the difference between natural or synthetic vitamins. Vitamin C is vitamin C whether it comes from citrus fruit or it is synthetically made. People who promote "natural" or "health" food are doing so to capitalize on the public's interest in good health. Normally you pay more. On the other hand, natural is not worse. All the research is not yet in and, therefore, it is certainly "O.K." to take natural vitamins rather than synthetic.

Fluids

The human body is made up of 50 percent to 70 percent water; therefore it is important to take in enough fluids daily. A good rule of thumb is to take in five to six glasses of water a day. Some of this liquid may be in the form of milk, soup, fruits, and vegetables but, it is best to get most of the fluids from water. You should drink enough fluids daily so that the urine becomes so diluted it is almost clear and colorless at least once during a twenty-four-hour period.

Many foods are good water sources. Some fruits and vegetables, such as tomatoes, eggplant, cauliflower, lettuce, strawberries, and watermelon, are over 90 percent water. Specifically, asparagus is 94 percent, green beans 92 percent, cabbage 92 percent, apples 85 percent, and oranges 86 percent. The amount of water you ingest daily will vary from five to six glasses in a normal day to an equivalent of ten to twelve on a hot day when you have exercised and lost body fluid through perspiration. You must be careful to ensure sufficient fluid replacement to prevent dehydration in such cases. Many of the commercial fluid replacement drinks are good because they also replace electrolytes (minerals) the body has lost through perspiration.

There are fluids to avoid just as there are foods to avoid. Caffeine-containing drinks such as coffee, tea, and colas should be eliminated or the amount decreased significantly. Caffeine-containing beverages have a strong effect on the body. Caffeine impairs motor coordination and reduces accuracy. Excess amounts can increase heart rate, stimulate the formation of acid-pepsin digestive juices in the stomach, and relate to fibrocystic breast disease in women. Caffeine is also a diuretic. A cup of coffee contains one hundred to one hundred fifty milligrams of caffeine. A cup of tea contains fifty to seventy-five milligrams, a twelve-ounce cola contains sixty milligrams, and a cup of hot chocolate about fifty milligrams.

Whole milk should be eliminated or the amount significantly reduced because of the excess fat contained in it. Most soft drinks should be de-emphasized because of the high-sugar, empty-calorie content. And without question, alcoholic beverages should be eliminated.

What's left? Try skim milk; it's refreshing. Unsweetened fruit juices are delicious and full of vitamins and minerals. If possible, replace the juices with the fresh fruit which will not only be thirst quenching but will also provide important fiber to the diet. Special drinks made with fruits, milk, and ice are tasty and nutritious.

Steps You Could Take

1. Take a one-a-day multivitamin-mineral supplement as insurance against a diet that may be lacking all the necessary vitamins and minerals.

2. If you feel a cold coming on, take extra vitamin C.

3. Limit caffeine intake to less then two hundred milligrams a day (maximum of two cups of coffee).

4. Ingest plenty of fluids every day. Fluids to emphasize are water, skim milk, fruit juices, and soft drinks without caffeine and sugar (one a day maximum). Fluids to de-emphasize are alcohol, whole milk, soft drinks with caffeine and sugar, tea, and coffee.

17

Putting It All Together

Purchasing and Preparing Food

Purchasing and preparing food are two important aspects of good nutrition. Remember a few basic rules when you go grocery shopping. Spend most of your time in the fresh produce section. Most of your caloric intake should come from fresh, whole foods, not processed ones. Buy fruits and vegetables that are in season and plan your meals around them. Recipes for delicious meatless dishes using vegetables and rice are plentiful. You can buy many of your fruits and vegetables from local vegetable markets, which would ensure freshness.

When you choose meats, think of poultry and fish. Many grocery stores have fresh fish, both freshwater and ocean varieties. Chicken is always an economical buy, and there are numerous appetizing ways to prepare it. Both chicken and fish, properly prepared, provide a dish high in protein but low in fat.

Become a label reader. Don't be confused by the words *fortified* and *enriched*. Most of these products have been stripped of most of their vitamins and minerals and then had a handful of nutrients restored. Emphasize brown rice over white rice, since brown rice has not been refined. Buy cereals with as much of the whole grain in them as possible. Read the nutritional breakdown on the box. Notice the fiber content; the cereal should have some fiber. Look at the complex carbohydrate and sugar content. It should be high in complex carbohydrates and low in sugar. Notice bread ingredients. Some breads may claim to contain whole-wheat flour and look brown but may just have a caramel coloring. Look for ingredients such as wheat bran, wheat germ, wheat berries, or perhaps a combination of grains such as rye, barley, or oats. The coarser and grainier the bread, the better. The only breads that are truly whole wheat will state "100 percent whole wheat."

When you prepare foods, peel and trim as little as possible. Raw fruits and vegetables keep vitamins and minerals that are in and close to the skins of those foods. If you plan to cook the fruit or vegetable, scrub it immediately prior to cooking but do not soak it. Cook as briefly as possible and serve immediately.

Several methods for cooking vegetables help retain many vitamins and minerals. For waterless cooking, several good brands of waterless cookware are on the market. The steaming method requires only a special metal basket placed inside a pan with a close-fitting lid. The food is cooked quickly, so that vitamins and minerals are not lost. Microwave cooking of vegetables is also good because little water is used.

As poultry and fish become more important in your daily diet, you need to remember a few tips. Skin the poultry. If you must fry the chicken, at least you're eliminating all the fat in the skin. A better method is to bake or broil the chicken, stir fry it, boil it, or use it in salads and casseroles. Fish is also healthier for you if it is broiled or baked. Experiment with various recipes and seasonings to find something just as tasty as the fried chicken or fish.

Several other practices will help you maintain a healthful eating style. Use vegetable oils instead of solid shortening not only in frying but also in baking. For instance, if a cookie recipe calls for one cup of butter, use half oil and half margarine. When you use eggs in cookies, cakes, or breads, normally leave out the yolks and substitute two whites for each whole egg. This way you can cut down on your cholesterol intake since the egg yolk is a high source of cholesterol. The sugar called for in *most* recipes can be cut by one-third to one-half and not affect the taste or texture. Think of all the calories that could be saved! To increase the fiber in your diet, bran and wheat germ can be mixed in or sprinkled on most foods without affecting taste or texture. Try sprinkling a tablespoon of wheat germ on your cereal in the morning or on vegetables and casseroles. Put it in orange juice! Bran is great in muffins and breads. Use your imagination.

According to the guidelines of Table 17.1, if an adult weighed seventy kilograms (154 pounds), he should consume 70 grams of protein and perhaps 35 to 40 grams of fat if he had a two thousand calorie intake per day. The choices he makes can have a fantastic difference in his balance of fats, carbohydrates, and proteins. The following table compares a traditional to a healthy day's diet. The healthy diet not only has about half the calories of the traditional but has much less fat (19 grams versus 190 grams) and an ample supply of protein.

TABLE 17.1
Daily Need for
Carbohydrates, Fats, and Proteins

NUTRIENT	DAILY REQUIREMENT
Protein	1. Adult: 1 gram per kilogram of body weight 2. Athlete, weightlifter, pregnant woman: 1 gram per kilogram of body weight plus 20 to 30 grams extra 3. Infant, growing teen-ager: 2 grams per kilogram of body weight
Fat	*20 to 30 grams* per day for a person on a 1000 calorie intake per day to a maximum of *50 to 60 grams* per day for a person on a 3000 or more calorie intake per day
Carbohydrates	Once you have achieved the minimum protein requirement and have stayed under the maximum fat allowance, all the remaining calories should come from carbohydrates—primarily complex.

The Basic Four Food Groups

Perhaps the simplest way to eat the recommended daily amount of carbohydrates, fats, proteins, vitamins, and minerals is to eat the recommended number of servings from each of the four groups.

Group one: fruits and vegetables. Every day you should have at least four servings from this group. An example of a serving would be one

TABLE 17.2
Comparison of Three Traditional
and Three Healthy Meals

FOOD	CALORIES	PROTEIN (GRAMS)	FAT (GRAMS)
BREAKFAST—TRADITIONAL			
2 fried eggs	170	10	12
2 bacon strips	170	4	8
1 cup hash browns	345	3	18
Toast with margarine	105	2	5
1/2 cup orange juice	60	2	0
1 cup whole milk	150	8	8
	1000	29	51

FOOD	CALORIES	PROTEIN (GRAMS)	FAT (GRAMS)
BREAKFAST—HEALTHY			
1 cup 40% Bran Flakes	105	4	1
½ banana	50	1	0
½ cup skim milk	43	4	0
1 slice wheat toast	60	3	1
1 tbsp. jelly	50	0	0
½ cup orange juice	60	2	0
1 cup skim milk	85	8	1
	453	22	3
LUNCH—TRADITIONAL			
¼ lb. hamburger	424	24	22
Regular fries	220	3	12
Chocolate shake	383	10	9
Apple pie	253	2	14
	1280	39	57
LUNCH—HEALTHY			
Tuna sandwich			
½ can water-packed tuna	100	22	1
2 wheat bread slices	150	5	2
½ cup lettuce	2	0	0
½ tomato	13	1	0
1 tbsp. W.W.* mayonnaise	40	0	4
1 cup skim milk	90	8	1
1 apple	80	0	1
4 oz. W.W.* cottage cheese	100	16	2
	575	52	11

*W.W. = Weight Watchers

FOOD	CALORIES	PROTEIN (GRAMS)	FAT (GRAMS)
DINNER—TRADITIONAL			
3 oz. roast beef	375	17	33
Baked potato with margarine	245	4	12
Canned buttered corn	140	4	1
Roll and margarine	120	2	6
Apple pie and ice cream	480	5	22
1 cup whole milk	150	8	8
	1510	40	82

FOOD	CALORIES	PROTEIN (GRAMS)	FAT (GRAMS)
DINNER—HEALTHY			
¼ broiled chicken	120	21	3
Baked potato (plain)	145	4	0
2 RyKrisp	88	2	0
1 cup fresh green beans	30	2	0
Angel food cake	135	3	0
1 cup sugared strawberries	100	1	1
1 cup skim milk	85	8	1
	703	41	5

SUMMARY FOR DAY

TRADITIONAL			
Breakfast	1000	29	51
Lunch	1280	39	57
Dinner	1510	40	82
Total	3790	108	190

HEALTHY			
Breakfast	453	22	3
Lunch	575	52	11
Dinner	703	41	5
Total	1731	115	19

whole fruit (banana, orange, apple, etc.), one-half cantaloupe or grapefruit, one slice of watermelon, one-half cup of most vegetables and berries, six ounces of fruit juice, one potato, or one small salad.

The best of this group would be raw fruits and vegetables, unsweetened juices, and potatoes (baked, regular or sweet). Cooked vegetables and canned fruits are acceptable.

Group two: grains in breads and cereals. Every day you should have at least four servings from this group. A serving would be one slice of bread, one ounce of cereal, or one-half cup of rice.

The best choices in this group would be 100 percent whole-grain breads, brown rice, and cereals as described earlier. Acceptable foods are crackers, white rice, pizza, macaroni, and waffles.

Group three: milk and milk products. You should have two daily servings from this group. A serving would be eight ounces of milk, eight ounces of yogurt, one-half cup of cottage cheese, or one-inch cube of cheese.

The best of this group would be skim milk, low-fat yogurt, and low-fat cheese. Two percent milk and ice milk are acceptable. The simplest way to achieve the requirement in this group is to have two glasses of skim milk a day. That is all an adult needs. Any more from this group adds unnecessary fat to the diet.

Group four: meat and protein. You should have two daily servings from this group. A serving would be two to three ounces of meat, two egg whites, one-half cup of legumes, one-half cup of nuts or seeds, or two tablespoons of peanut butter.

The best sources for this group would be roasted chicken or turkey, fish, egg whites, and legumes such as lentils, peas, or beans. Whole eggs, lean beef, seeds, and nuts are acceptable. Because of the high fat content, the following foods in this group are to be avoided: fish sticks, commercially prepared chicken, egg and cheese dishes, bacon, cold cuts, and frankfurters.

Eat Well-balanced Meals

People today tend to skip meals, especially breakfast. Lack of time is the usual excuse, but it's important to eat balanced meals each day. Decide how many calories you need to consume each day to lose, maintain, or gain weight, depending on your situation. Determine what 30 percent of those calories would be and let that be the amount you have for each meal: breakfast, lunch, and dinner. The remaining 10 percent may be divided up into snacks—midmorning, midafternoon, or evening. Whatever you do, don't wait until evening to consume all your calories since it appears that food eaten after 2:00 P.M. tends to stay in and on your body longer. Eating most of your calories before 2:00 P.M. gives your body more hours to digest and burn them.

The following examples are suggestions for what one day of meals, including snacks, might look like:

Breakfast
6 ounces orange juice, or 1 whole orange
Bowl of high-fiber cereal (Note the cereals suggested in chap. 16 or make your own granola.)
Banana
1 slice 100% whole-wheat toast with jelly, no margarine or butter (If you are trying to lose weight, you may want to eliminate the toast and jelly.)
8 ounces skim milk

Lunch
Sandwich of tuna or chicken on 100% whole-wheat bread with lettuce or sprouts
Carrot and celery sticks
Fresh fruit (apple, pear, orange, etc.)
8 ounces skim milk
(Peanut butter could be substituted for meat, and a tossed salad could replace carrots and celery. Yogurt is also good. It is easy to make at home without all the added sugar of the ones made commercially. If you're trying to lose weight, have only half a sandwich.)

Dinner
4-6 ounces baked fish or chicken
1 medium baked potato or brown rice
$1/2$-$3/4$ cup fresh steamed broccoli or spinach salad
$1/2$-$3/4$ cup peas
Water
Piece of fresh fruit or fruit salad
(If you're trying to lose weight, cut down on portions, but eat all the foods above.)

Snacks and Desserts

Snacks and desserts don't have to be bad for you. Some suggestions for snacks include raw vegetables, fruit, cold cereals, and popcorn (unsalted and unbuttered). Raw nuts are good for you but only in limited quantities because they are high in fat and calories. If you crave something sweet, try dried fruits. Most grocery stores have raisins, dried apples, bananas, prunes, and so on. Here again you must limit the amount. Discipline in all areas is important.

Desserts don't have to be eliminated from the diet, only modified or decreased. Cutting your piece of dessert in half each day may save one hundred to three hundred calories. Take just enough so you don't feel deprived but you still satisfy your sweet tooth. Perhaps allow yourself a dessert only three days a week. The most important thing is that you control your will power. Experiment and see what is best for you. If you want to eliminate sugary desserts, try fruit.

Guidelines for Controlling Your Caloric Intake

1. Sit down to eat at the kitchen or dining room table. Get used to eating in one place. *Don't* eat in front of the TV, at your desk, at a movie, or

at an athletic contest. This alone could eliminate several hundred calories a day.

2. Eat only at specific times. You will be less likely to grab a snack when you think you're hungry or because someone else is eating.

3. Use a smaller plate when possible. A small plate that is filled can look as though you have a lot more food than you really do.

4. Eat slowly. Not only is this better for your digestion, but your appestat signals your brain that you're full before you've had a chance to stuff yourself.

5. Carry a calorie chart to help you learn the approximate number of calories in most of the foods you eat. Small books are available at grocery stores and bookstores that fit into a woman's purse or a man's suitcoat pocket.

6. Don't use food as a reward.

7. Make a shopping list when you buy food and stick to it. Don't buy on impulse.

8. Don't grocery shop when you're hungry.

9. Store food at home out of sight. Don't keep cookies and snacks on the counter.

10. Clear the table immediately after a meal.

11. Whenever possible, eat raw, unprocessed foods. For example, a potato costs about twelve cents per pound and contains no fat and little sodium. Potato chips, on the other hand, cost two dollars per pound and contain 65 percent fat and one hundred times the sodium of a potato.

12. Little things mean a lot. One snack or drink every day could add up to 36,500 calories in one year or about ten pounds. A daily half-hour walk could burn 67,700 calories in one year or eighteen pounds. Eliminating toast at breakfast could mean fifteen pounds in a year.

Steps You Could Take

1. Go back to chapters 14 and 15. Analyze your caloric expenditure on a daily basis.

2. Depending upon whether you want to gain weight, lose weight, or stay the same, plan a diet for seven days that includes the four basic food groups and emphasize the foods discussed in chapter 16. Remember, a 3500 caloric positive balance will add one pound and a 3500 caloric negative balance will lose one pound. Your caloric intake should be at least 1000 calories per day. Consult nutrition books to obtain the specific calories of the foods in your diet.

Part IV

Mental Attitude and
Emotional Health

18

The Mind and Health

Spirit, Body, and Mind

The human person has often been defined as having three basic components—spirit, body, and mind. The spirit is that part God activated within us when we became living creatures. The spirit within us seeks after God, righteousness, peace, health, happiness, and joy. If we are living as God would have us to live, the human spirit is energized by God, and the fruits of the Holy Spirit are abundant in our lives.

The body is the structure that houses the spirit and the mind. It is their servant. It receives sensory input from the ears, eyes, nose, mouth, skin, muscles, joints, and other body organs and sends it to the mind for interpretation and response.

The mind comprises intellect, emotion, and will. God created us with minds to think, emotions to feel, and freedom to choose. Hence, it is in the mind where the greatest struggles often take place and decisions are made whether to follow the urgings of the spirit or the impulses of the flesh.

It is important for us to note that these three components never operate independently; each of us functions as a total person. We do not bypass our minds, for example, as we walk in the spirit. Nor do we choose between following body or mind. We operate as total persons.

The Power of the Mind

Jim Thorpe, judged the greatest athlete of the first half of the twentieth century, used not only his great physical talents to perfection but also the powerful force of his mind. In the 1912 Olympics he won both the decathlon and pentathlon, truly one of the greatest records in the history of the Olympic games. Not only did he train hard physically, but he concentrated mentally on each event he was to perform.

Before he made the long jump, he measured out twenty-three feet, drew a line, sat down, and looked at the distance for ten to fifteen minutes. Then he closed his eyes and for twenty minutes pictured himself jumping twenty-three feet and going past the line. When the time came for him to jump, he won the event with a jump of twenty-three feet three inches! "For as he thinks in his heart, so is he" (Prov. 23:7). No by-passing the mind there!

Jim Thorpe's visualizing his body performing in a specific way has been scientifically documented to be effective. The concept is often called "mental practice." If you first learn the basics of an activity, then practice both physically and mentally, you will improve much faster than if you practice only physically. The most commonly recommended method of practicing mentally is go to a quiet area, close your eyes, and visualize in your mind your successful completion of the activity. Continue to visualize this again and again for fifteen minutes every day. It works!

Hypnosis is another example of the power of the mind—in this case the power of the subconscious part of the mind. A person who *allows* himself to be hypnotized may be told he is weak and can't pick up a pencil. When the person is brought out of the hypnotic spell and asked to lift a pencil, he will be unable to do it.

Studies on the electrical activity in the muscles reveal that the conscious centers of the brain will send nervous impulses to the muscles of the arm that are sufficient to lift the pencil. However, the power of the subconscious suggestion, "You can't lift the pencil," is so strong that the subconscious mind will also send impulses to other arm muscles to oppose the lifting of the pencil. So the person has a tremendous conflict with himself—one force, the conscious mind, attempting to lift the pencil, and another force, the subconscious, trying to prevent the lifting of the pencil.

Unfortunately, many people literally hypnotize themselves by what they think about themselves. It is not just what we express outwardly about ourselves, but what we feel deeply within that counts. Our minds play a definite role in our health. If we desire optimal health, we must begin to visualize it deep within our beings.

A woman had struggled for years to lose weight, but her weight loss followed the typical yo-yo pattern. Lose-gain-lose-gain ad infinitum. She would drop to 160 pounds, then go back up to 180, then down to 160, only to regain weight again. It seemed as if she could never go below

160. This went on for more than four years. Could it be that she subconsciously pictured herself at 160?

I suggested to her that she picture herself at 130 (which would be her ideal weight) and that every day she quietly meditate fifteen minutes and see herself at 130 pounds in a size nine dress or in a flattering swimsuit. After several months, it worked. She began to drop below 160, and finally she did reach 130. Because her body, mind, and spirit all worked together, she pictured herself at that weight, her mind took control of her behavior, she worked toward that weight, and she stayed there!

Maxwell Maltz, M.D., in his book *Psycho-Cybernetics*, writes that within each of us is a power working toward health, happiness, peace, and success. But we can choose to inhibit this power through anxiety, fear, and self-condemnation and suffer the negative effects of these emotions. In order to harness the positive force within ourselves we must think positively and imagine ourselves healthy, happy, peaceful, and successful.

Control Your Thoughts

The Scriptures repeatedly admonish us to control our thoughts and to think positively in order to please God and to have a happy, joyous life. In order to control our thoughts, we must allow the Spirit to control our minds. If we do that, the results will be love, joy, peace, patience, kindness, goodness, faithfulness, gentleness, and self-control (see Gal. 5:22–23). If we possessed all these qualities, we would certainly have an abundant life.

These fruits do not happen by mere wishing. We are to think good, wholesome thoughts (see Phil. 4:8). As thoughts enter our minds, we are to evaluate them in accordance with God's Word (see 2 Cor. 10:5). The tendency too often is to think of the negative, dwell on the problems, and focus on the aches and pains. If anyone dwells too long on negative thoughts, the subconscious will begin to take control and paralyze the conscious mind. The body will react, and sickness and depression can result (see chap. 19).

Turn Negative Thoughts Into Positive Thoughts

NEGATIVE THOUGHT	POSITIVE THOUGHT
I can't do it.	"I can do all things through Christ who strengthens me" (Phil. 4:13). All things are possible because I believe (see Mark 9:23).
I have difficulty taking charge.	God has told me to take dominion over all living things, including myself. I will take dominion over myself (see Gen. 1:28).

NEGATIVE THOUGHT	POSITIVE THOUGHT
I'm sick.	I'm healed and whole (see Isa. 53:5; 1 Pet. 2:24). I'll get my health back (see Jer. 30:17).
I'm afraid.	"God has not given us a spirit of fear, but of power and of love and of a sound mind" (2 Tim. 1:7). God is with me, He will strengthen me (see Isa. 41:10).
I'm weak.	The Lord is the strength of my life (see Ps. 27:1). Because I know God, I will display strength and take action (see Dan. 11:32).
I'm worried and frustrated.	I will cast all my cares on Him because He cares for me (see 1 Pet. 5:7).
Satan is always tempting me.	Greater is He who is in me than he who is in the world (see 1 John 4:4).
I'm depressed.	In God's presence I have fullness of joy (see Ps. 16:11). The joy of the Lord is my strength (see Neh. 8:10).
I have difficulty controlling my diet and exercise habits.	I have complete control of my body and make it a slave (see 1 Cor. 9:27). I am a conqueror (see Rom. 8:37).

Negative thoughts will come to all of us. The challenge is to capture them, control them, evaluate them, and turn them into a personal, positive response. Then meditate on the positive response. We should repeat the positive statement many times every day until the positive is so much a part of our conscious thoughts that it is driven into our subconscious minds; then we will have won the battle. The body will begin to react according to the positive thoughts.

Controlling our thoughts is imperative for good health. If we fail, negative thoughts will lead to emotions of defeat, anxiety, distress, and depression, and these emotions can spark many health problems.

Steps You Could Take

1. Meditation on God's Word results in our being as solid and strong as a tree (see Ps. 1:1–3). Therefore, meditate on God's Word daily. Fix your meditation on the positive aspects of the Scriptures.

2. Visualize yourself as a healthy, disciplined exerciser, at the weight you desire, and as a person who controls food and is not controlled by it.

19

Emotions and Health

Stress and Emotions

We all live in environments that place varying degrees of stress upon us every day and to which we may respond in different ways. If we make decisions guided by the Holy Spirit, positive emotions result that lead to optimal health and happiness. If we make decisions guided by the flesh, negative emotions result that lead to poor health and depression.

For example, your boss walks past you in the morning and neglects to say hello. How might you respond? Perhaps with fear: "He is going to fire me!" or "What did I do wrong this time?" Perhaps with anger: "I'm getting upset with his ignoring me in the morning!" or "Who does he think he is?" Perhaps with resentment, jealousy, or bitterness: "I wish I was the boss so I could do as I please," or "Life just isn't fair!"

All these emotions are negative and cause the body to respond in a harmful way. The adrenal glands will release chemicals known as catecholamines, such as adrenalin, that cause increased heart rate, blood sugar, blood fats, blood pressure, respiratory rate, and perspiration; irregular heartbeats; shortened blood-clotting time; and slowed digestive processes.

Just think of all the reactions that take place in your body immediately as the result of negative emotions! There are times when these reactions are essential. If you are walking alone and someone attempts to attack you, fear will initiate these responses that prepare the body for fight or flight. The extra burst of energy may be what was required to help you run away and save your life.

God made our bodies to respond to fear so we could physically respond to danger. God intends us to have fear only when we are in physical danger and need extra energy to escape. All these bodily reactions assist in a quick physical response. The shortened clotting time when we are cut or bruised protects us from excess bleeding. What wonderful bodies God has created with their emergency response mechanisms!

When fear and other adverse emotions affect our lives when they shouldn't, when we do not respond physically but instead brood, become anxious, and worry about a problem we perceive to be real, our bodies' reactions that were meant to protect us have the potential of causing damage. If the negative emotions are allowed to continue unchecked for weeks and months, they can lead to high blood pressure, stroke, heart attack, ulcers, migraines, colitis, skin disorders, allergies, asthma, arthritis, or depression. Even cancer has been associated with long-term negative emotions.

Stress alone is not the culprit that causes disease. It is an inescapable part of living. Stress itself is not positive or negative, but the way we respond to stress is critical. When a person is asked out on a date, stress is placed on the person. The person can respond positively with joy, happiness, and excitement or negatively with fear, worry, and anxiety.

Marriage, childbirth, the departure of a young person for college, a new job in a new city, and retirement are all examples of stressful situations. Each has the potential of producing positive emotions within a person that can contribute to optimal health and well-being. Or the stress can elicit negative emotions that persist week after week and month after month, slowly draining the body of its energy and its ability to resist disease. Eventually symptoms of disease develop and the disease itself may occur. Now the disease is real, not imaginary; it was allowed to take hold of the body because of long-lasting negative emotions.

Symptoms of Negative Emotions

Often the results of poorly handled stress are obvious, and we realize what is happening to us. We feel tense, our hands are cold and clammy, and we have trouble sleeping at night. Recognizing that our bodies are not responding satisfactorily to stress is the beginning of overcoming negative emotions and handling the stress better the next time.

One evening I was describing to Donna a situation that bothered me. As I related the situation to her, I could feel myself reliving the situation and becoming tense. I stopped and asked her to get the blood-pressure cuff and check my blood pressure. Both systolic and diastolic pressures were up. I closed my eyes, focused my attention on a peaceful scene, and relaxed. Within three minutes my blood pressure dropped to normal. I have learned to be aware of tenseness, to overcome it, and to relax.

Too often, however, when stress is handled poorly over a long time, we become unaware of our bodies' reactions. Often emotional conflicts are difficult to accept so we suppress feelings and are no longer consciously aware of them. Prolonged, suppressed negative emotions play a dominant role in many physical ailments. An individual goes from doctor to doctor, treatment to treatment, medicine to medicine, prayer to prayer, but the healing of the physical ailment doesn't occur. The reason for the failure of both prayer and medicine is that the physical problem will not go away until the emotional problem that led to it is cured.

One of the most important things you can do when you have a physical ailment that does not respond well to either medicine or prayer is to examine your emotions. Is there bitterness, worry, fear, guilt, self-pity, anger, or any other negative emotion that you may have suppressed? If you answer yes or perhaps, there is a way to change your negative emotions for positive ones.

TABLE 19.1
Summary of Stress Symptoms

Pounding of the heart	Irritability
Depression	Inability to concentrate
Dizziness	Fatigue
Tension	Nervous tic
Trembling	Grinding of the teeth
Insomnia	Sweating
Pain in the neck	Pain in the low back

Overcoming Negative Emotions

Since we live in a world where stress is inescapable, it is vital that we learn how to successfully manage the stress we face and prevent negative emotions from developing. We have some suggestions to help you manage stress.

1. *Exercise.* We have described how the negative emotions of fear, worry, and anger prepare the body for a physical response by releasing adrenalin into the blood stream. Sometimes a hectic and busy day can produce the same effects. To prevent the harmful side effects of excess adrenalin on the body, one of the easiest and most readily available curatives is exercise. Since God created us to respond to stress physically, exercise is obviously His remedy for stress. Rather than vent anger or frustration at someone else, try exercise. In this way tension is released in an acceptable way and health is enhanced. Many business executives conduct their exercise program at 5:00 or 6:00 P.M. after a busy day of work to help relieve the tensions of the day. The exercise should be aerobic as described in earlier chapters.

Exercise can also be beneficial in the treatment of depression. Therapists are beginning to prescribe exercise, primarily jogging, as a therapeutic mode to treat depressed patients. The results have been excellent. Therefore, exercise provides both physiological and psychological benefits.

2. *Replace fear with faith.* Fear of physical danger can be beneficial and give us the extra physical energy we need to escape. Too often, however, fear is not of a physical danger but of some situation, person, or task. Fear of failure is not unusual. This type of fear is deadly to the body because rather than a physical response, the common response is lethargy.

Fear that is not God-given must be faced head-on and conquered. If it is allowed to remain, that which is greatly feared will come upon us (see Job 3:25). The Scriptures frequently tell us to "fear not." We must replace fear with faith. Fear tells us, "I can't do it." Faith tells us, "I can do it" (see Phil. 4:13). Faith does not just happen: "Faith comes by hearing, and hearing by the word of God" (Rom. 10:17).

Fear can be overtaken by faith. As we study and meditate on God's Word and allow our minds to be fixed on Christ, fear will leave, and faith and peace will enter. But remember, faith without action is of no value (see James 2:26). As we increase the faith in our hearts, we must attack fears and conquer them. We should analyze and list the fears. Then one by one, attack and conquer them until they are all gone. I have seen many students at ORU with a fear of water. What a joy it has been to see them over the weeks and months gradually overcome that fear and learn to swim. As fear is conquered, the opportunity for optimal health increases.

3. *Replace bitterness with forgiveness and joy.* The Scriptures teach us to "watch out that no bitterness takes root among you, for as it springs up it causes deep trouble, hurting many in their spiritual lives" (Heb. 12:15 TLB). Bitterness is often the result of suffering a hurt, either real or perceived. Rather than respond with forgiveness, we harbor the feelings, and a root of bitterness springs up that affects us spiritually and physically. In the book of Proverbs we read that "a crushed spirit dries up the bones" (17:22 NIV) and "envy rots the bones" (14:30 NIV). On the basis of these passages, some authorities have associated arthritis with negative emotions.

Bitterness leads not only to problems with the bones but to a weakened body and a reduced resistance to various diseases and health problems. "When I kept silent about my sin, my body wasted away/...My vitality was drained away" (Ps. 32:3–4 NASB). Conflict in a marriage that leads to bitterness can cause health problems in the mates (see Prov. 12:4).

To replace bitterness we must make a choice to forgive those who have wronged us. Jesus emphasized that we need to forgive "seventy times seven" (Matt. 18:22) and that if we don't forgive others, we are asking God not to forgive us (see Matt. 6:12–15; Mark 11:25–26). In Ephesians we read, "Be as ready to forgive others as God for Christ's sake has forgiven you" (4:32 PHILLIPS). We must learn to accept that many situations are out of our control. We should look for the good in others and in every situation since "in all things God works for the good" (Rom. 8:28 NIV).

Put joy in your heart. It is good medicine (see Prov. 17:22)! "A tranquil heart is life to the body" (Prov. 14:30 NASB). A number of research studies have reported that happy people live healthier and longer lives, regardless of their other health habits. Allow the joy of the Lord to be your strength (see Neh. 8:10).

4. *Replace negative emotions with fruits of the Spirit.* Fear and bitterness are two emotions that seem to be especially prevalent and need specific attention. Other emotions also need to be replaced with positive forces so we can have optimal healthy lives. When stresses face us in various areas, we must respond from the Spirit rather than the flesh. Responses of the Spirit include hope, generosity, love, empathy, and patience while responses of the flesh include worry, selfishness, hate, criticism, and anger.

Steps You Could Take

1. Exercise aerobically for at least thirty minutes each day (preferably late afternoon) to help relieve the tension caused by stress.

2. Become sensitive to what your body is telling you. If you feel tense, close your eyes, lean back in your chair, and relax for five to ten minutes. Let your mind think of positive and peaceful experiences, and feel the tension leave your body.

3. If you struggle with negative emotions, meditate on God's Word and replace fear with faith, worry with hope, bitterness with forgiveness, hate with love, anger with patience, criticism with empathy, and selfishness with generosity.

4. Be happy, laugh, and look for the good in others.

Finally, brethren, whatever is true, whatever is honorable, whatever is right, whatever is pure, whatever is lovely, whatever is of good repute, if there is any excellence and if anything worthy of praise, let your mind dwell on these things....and the God of peace shall be with you (Phil. 4:8–9 NASB).

20

Sowing and Reaping

Sometimes it seems as though the results we seek don't occur. We exercise, we diet, we work at thinking positive thoughts and controlling our negative emotions, and we pray; yet we don't lose the weight as rapidly as we would like or we don't improve our health as quickly as we had thought we would. We are tempted to give up. We should remember to "not grow weary while doing good, for in due season we shall reap if we do not lose heart" (Gal. 6:9).

Patience

Don't give up! Do not grow weary of doing what is right! We have outlined in this book an approach to optimal health and fitness that is consistent with God's spiritual and natural laws. If you live your life according to these laws, they will work, but you have to be patient. Don't expect results overnight. Any program that promises instant success is quackery. God didn't create us that way. All of God's creation was created in accordance with the sowing and reaping principle: "Do not be deceived, God is not mocked; for whatever a man sows, this he will also reap" (Gal. 6:7 NASB).

To become healthy and fit requires more than wishing. It requires the planting of good seed. The process of planting good seeds for health involves an aerobic exercise program (chaps. 8 and 9), a muscle-building program (chap. 10), a good, nutritional diet- and weight-control program (chaps. 16 and 17), a vision for health (chap. 18), and the control of negative emotions (chap. 19).

For the seed to grow and produce results requires time and patience and, most of all, consistency. God promised Abraham a son (see Gen. 15). Fulfillment of that promise took some twenty-five years. During those years, until Isaac was born, Abraham "did not waver....but was strengthened in faith" (Rom. 4:20). He was patient, and he did not give up.

The same was true for Joseph. In his teen-age years he saw a vision of his brothers bowing down to him. Yet it was more than twenty years later that the vision came true. Throughout that time, Joseph was faithful amidst his many trials (see Gen. 37–45). When you know you are visualizing the will of God, do not grow weary while doing good.

Realistic Goals

Perhaps one reason some people become weary in doing good is that they set their goals too high and attempt to accomplish too much too soon. If you have been struggling with an exercise program, weight control, a good diet, and control of your emotions, perhaps you should work on changing only one or two lifestyle patterns at a time rather than attempting several at once. In this way, you can bring all your lifestyle patterns in line with God's natural and spiritual laws.

Give to Others

Sometimes individuals become so concerned about themselves they fail to look beyond their own problems. If you become too self-centered and pity yourself because you have failed to conquer your problem, chances are you will never conquer it. Often, to solve your own problem, you will need to plant some good seeds with other persons who are struggling with the same problem you have.

For example, if you are struggling to lose weight, in addition to exercising and eating the right foods, you should help someone else who is struggling with the same problem. Plant a good seed in someone else and expect a harvest for yourself. As you encourage another person, you help yourself.

Job faced a multitude of difficulties. He lost his family, his fortunes, and his health. Throughout most of the book of Job he wondered why all the calamities descended on him but "the LORD restored the fortunes of Job when he prayed for his friends" (42:10 NASB). Jesus said, "Give, and it will be given to you" (Luke 6:38).

In Isaiah 58:1–11 is a picture of God's view of how to solve problems. Verses 1 to 6 reveal man trying hard to solve his problem through fasting and prayer. But God says that this is not enough: you should (1) give to the hungry, (2) take care of the homeless, (3) clothe the naked, and (4) take care of your relatives (v. 7). Then you can expect health (v. 9) and strength to your bones (v. 11).

What Is Your Real Desire?

Perhaps another reason that changes in your health and fitness don't occur is that you are not really serious about making the change. You may talk of your good intentions, read about all the new approaches to fitness, and try various exercises and diets. But the Scriptures teach that "you will know them by their fruits" (Matt. 7:16). Improved fitness and weight control are the fruits of a sincere desire that leads to a consistent, positive lifestyle. Wishes and enthusiasm will not produce lasting changes. So, if you have been attempting to change your lifestyle to a healthier one and have not succeeded, perhaps you should evaluate your desire. Do you want to change badly enough?

A Way of Living

As you lay this book aside, I challenge you to commit yourself to a whole new lifestyle. This is not a quick fix or an easy way to health. It involves discipline and dedication of your total being. It requires a life-style of meditation on the Scriptures, aerobic and muscle-development exercises, weight control, good nutrition, and a positive mental attitude.

The benefits far outweigh the efforts. Excellent health, happiness, joy, peace, long life, and oneness with your Creator can be yours. You can do it! Set realistic goals. Be consistent. Have patience. "Let us lay aside every weight, and the sin which so easily ensnares us, and let us run with endurance the race that is set before us" (Heb. 12:1).

Appendix

Marathon Training Schedule

1. This schedule presumes that you are currently training at least thirty miles per week. If you are running less, don't start this training schedule until you are regularly running at that level.
2. Begin the schedule three months before the marathon you want to run.
3. The days marked with an asterisk (*) are the days when you should run at a faster pace than you plan to run the marathon.
4. On all other days you should run at about the pace you plan to run the marathon.

Day	Week 1	Week 2	Week 3	Week 4	Week 5	Week 6
1	4	4	5	5	5	5
2	6	7	8	8	8	10
3	3*	3*	3*	4*	4*	4*
4	6	7	7	8	8	8
5	4*	4*	4*	4*	5*	5*
6	9	10	11	12	14	15
7	Rest	Rest	Rest	Rest	Rest	Rest
Total	32	35	38	41	44	47

Day	Week 7	Week 8	Week 9	Week 10	Week 11	Week 12
1	6	6	8	8	10	10
2	4*	5*	6*	6*	7*	5*
3	10	10	10	10	10	7
4	5*	5*	5*	6*	6*	4
5	9	9	9	9	9	Rest
6	16	18	18	21	18	Marathon
7	Rest	Rest	Rest	Rest	Rest	
Total	50	53	56	60	60	

Day	Week 1	Week 2	Week 3	Week 4	Week 5	Week 6
1	4	4	5	5 Rest	5 Bike	5 Bike
2	6	7	8	8 5	8	10
3	3*	3*	3*	4*6	4*	4* 5
4	6	7	7	8	8	8 5
5	4*	4*	4*	4*	5*	5*
6	9	10	11 12	12 13	14	15 16
7	Rest	Rest	Rest	Rest	Rest	Rest
Total	32	35	38	41	44	47

Day	Week 7	Week 8	Week 9	Week 10	Week 11	Week 12
1	6 Rest	6	8	8	10	10
2	4* 6	5*	6*	6*	7*	5*
3	10	10 12	10	10	10	7
4	5* 6	5* 2	5*	6*	6*	4
5	9 6	9 5	9	9	9	Rest
6	16	18	18 22	21 18	18 15	Marathon
7	Rest	Rest	Rest	Rest	Rest	
Total	50	53	56	60	60	

Bibliography

Books

Ardell, Donald B. *High-Level Wellness*. Emmaus, Penn: Rodale Press, 1977.
Bailey, Covert. *Fit or Fat*. Boston: Houghton Mifflin Company, 1978.
Brand, Paul, and Philip Yancey. *Fearfully and Wonderfully Made*. Grand Rapids, Mich.: Zondervan Publishing House, 1981.
Chapian, Marie. *Free to Be Thin*. Minneapolis: Bethany House Publishers, 1979.
Comfort, Alex. *The Process of Aging*. New York: New American Library, 1964.
Cooper, Kenneth H. *The Aerobics Way*. New York: Bantam Books, Inc., 1978.
Couey, Dick. *Building God's Temple*. Minneapolis: Burgess Publishing Company, 1982.
DeBakey, Michael, and Antonio Gotto. *The Living Heart*. New York: Grosset & Dunlap, 1977.
Fixx, James. *The Complete Book of Running*. New York: Random House, 1977.
Gallup, George, and Evan Hill. *The Secrets of Long Life*. New York: Random House, 1960.
Galton, Lawrence. *How Long Will I Live*. New York: Macmillan Publishing Co., 1976.
Hafen, Brent Q. *Nutrition, Food & Weight Control*. Newton, Mass.: Allyn & Bacon, 1981.
Heller, A. L. *Your Body, His Temple*. Nashville: Thomas Nelson Publishers, 1981.
Jones, Billy M. *Health-Seekers in the Southwest, 1817–1900*. Norman: University of Oklahoma Press, 1967.
Kostrubala, Thaddeus. *The Joy of Running*. New York: Pocket Books, Inc., 1976.
Kraus, Hans. *The Cause, Prevention, and Treatment of Backache, Stress and Tension*. New York: Simon & Schuster, 1965.
Kraus, Hans, and Wilhelm Raab. *Hypolinetic Disease*. Springfield, Ill.: Charles C. Thomas, 1961.

Kugler, Hans. *Slowing Down the Aging Process*. New York: Pyramid, 1973.

Kurtzman, Joel, and Phillip Gordon. *No More Dying*. Los Angeles: J. P. Tarcher, 1976.

Leonard, Jon N., J. L. Hofer, and N. Pritikin. *Live Longer Now: The First One Hundred Years of Your Life*. New York: Grosset & Dunlap, 1974.

McMillen, S. I. *None of These Diseases*. Old Tappan, N.J.: Fleming H. Revell Co., 1974.

Miller, Jonas. *Prescription for Total Health and Longevity*. South Plainfield, N.J.: Bridge Publishers, 1979.

Oehm, Rudolph. *The Joy of Good Health*. Eugene, Oreg.: Harvest House Publishers, 1980.

Roberts, Oral. *Seven Divine Aids For Your Healing and Health*. Tulsa: Oral Roberts University, 1965.

Root, Leon, and Thomas Kiernan. *Oh, My Aching Back!* New York: New American Library, 1975.

Shedd, Charles W. *The Fat Is in Your Head*. Waco, Tex.: Word Books, 1972.

Articles

Bray, A. S. "The Overweight Patient." *Archives of Internal Medicine* 5 (1976): 276–308.

Brownell, K. D., et al. "Physical Activity in the Development and Control of Obesity." *Obesity* (1980).

Byrne, Jean T. et al. "In Sickness and in Health: The Effects of Religion." *Health Education* (January/February 1979): 6–10.

Cassel, J. et al. "Occupation and Physical Activity and Coronary Heart Disease." *Archives of Internal Medicine* 128 (1971): 920–28.

Chlouverakis, C. "Dietary and Medical Treatments of Obesity: An Evaluative Review." *Addictive Behavior* 1 (1975): 3–12.

Cooper, K. H., et al. "Physical Fitness Levels and Selected Coronary Risk Factors. A Crossectional Study." *Journal of American Medical Association* 236 (1976): 66.

Dahlkoetter, JoAnn, et al. "Obesity and the Unbalanced Energy Equation: Exercise Versus Eating Habit Change." *Journal of Consulting and Clinical Psychology* 47 (1979): 898–905.

Drenick, Ernst J., et al. "Excessive Mortality and Causes of Death in Morbidly Obese Men." *Journal of American Medical Association* (February 1, 1980): 443–45.

Dressendorfer, Rudolph H. "Physiological Profile of a Masters Runner." *The Physician and Sportsmedicine* 8 (August 1980): 49–52.

Dublin, L. I. "Relation of Obesity to Longevity." *The New England Journal of Medicine* 248 (1953): 971.

Dwyer, Terry, et al. "A Comparison of Trends of Coronary Heart Disease Mortality in Australia, USA, England, and Wales with Reference to Three Major Risk Factors—Hypertension, Cigarette Smoking, and Diet." *International Journal of Epidemiology* 9 (1980): 65–71.

Enger, S. Chr., et al. "High Density Lipoprotein (HPL) and Physical Activity." *Scandinavian Journal of Clinical Laboratory Investigation* 37 (1977): 251.

Enstrom, James E. "Cancer Mortality Among Mormons in California During 1968–1975." *Journal of Clinical Investigation* 65 (November 1980): 1073–82.

Epstein, L. H., et al. "Behavioral Contracting: Health Behaviors." *Clinical Behavior Therapy Review* 1 (1979): 1–22.

————. "Aerobic Exercise and Weight." *Addictive Behaviors* 5 (1980): 371–88.

————. "A Nutritionally Based School Program for Control of Eating in Obese Children." *Behavior Therapy* 9 (1978): 766–88.

————. "A Comparison of Lifestyle Change and Programmed Aerobic Exercise on Weight and Fitness Changes in Obese Children." *Behavior Therapy* 13 (1982): 651–65.

————. "Child and Parent Weight Loss in Family-Based Behavior Modification Program." *Journal of Consulting and Clinical Psychology* 49 (1981): 675–85.

————. "Comparison of Family-Based Behavior Modification and Nutrition Education for Childhood Obesity." *Journal of Pediatric Psychology* 5 (1980): 25–36.

————. "The Effects of Contract and Lottery Procedures on Attendance and Fitness in Aerobic Exercise." *Behavior Modification* 4 (1980): 465–80.

Erikssen, Jan et al. "Coronary Risk Factors and Physical Fitness in Healthy Middle-Aged Men." *Acta Medical Scandinavica* 645 (1981): 57–64.

Friedman, Bonnie Jones, et al. "Running for Life, Health, and Pleasure." *American Journal of Nursing* 78 (April 1978): 602–7.

Froehlicher, Victor F. "Does Exercise Conditioning Delay Progression of Myocardial Ischemia in Coronary Atherosclerotic Heart Disease?" *Cardiovascular Clinics* 8 (1977): 11.

————. "Does Exercise Protect from Coronary Artery Disease?" *Advanced Cardiology* 27 (1980): 237–42.

Graham, Thomas W., et al. "Frequency of Church Attendance and Blood Pressure Elevation." *Journal of Behavior Medicine* 1 (1978): 37–43.

Gwinup, G. "Effect of Exercise Alone on Weight of Obese Women." *Archives of Internal Medicine* 135 (1975): 676–80.

Gyntelberg, F., et al. "Blood Pressure Reduction by Change in Life Style: The CVD Intervention Study in Glostrup." *Acta Medica Scandinavica* 646 (1980): 10–14.

Harris, M. B. et al. "Self-Directed Weight Control Through Eating and Exercise." *Behavior Research and Therapy* 11 (1973): 523–29.

Hartung, Harley G. et al. "Relation of Diet to High-Density-Lipoprotein Cholesterol in Middle-aged Marathon Runners, Joggers, and Inactive Men." *The New England Journal of Medicine* 302 (1980): 357–61.

Hubert, Helen B. "Obesity as an Independent Risk Factor for Cardiovascular Disease: A 26-Year Follow-up of Participants in the Framingham Heart Study." *Circulation* 67 (May 1983): 968–76.

Kahn, H. A. "The Relationship of Reported Coronary Heart Disease Mortality to Physical Activity of Work." *American Journal of Public Health* 53 (1963): 1058–67.

Karronen, M. J., et al. "Heart Disease and Employment: Cardiovascular Studies on Lumberjacks." *Journal of Occupational Medicine* 3 (1961): 49–53.

Kent, Saul. "Diet and Increased Life Span." *Geriatrics* (July 1980): 101–3.

Keys, A., et al. "Indices of Relative Weight and Obesity." *Journal of Chronic Diseases* 25 (1972): 329–43.

_____ . "Epidemiological Studies Related to Coronary Heart Disease: Characterisitics of Men Aged 40–59 in Seven Countries." *Acta Medica Scandinavica* 450 (1966): 1–392.

King, Haitung, et al. "Cancer Mortality Among Chinese in the United States." *Journal of Clinical Investigation* 65 (November 1980).

_____ . "American White Protestant Clergy as a Low-Risk Population for Mortality Research." *Journal of Clinical Investigation* 65 (November 1980).

Kramsch, Dieter M. et al. "Reduction of Coronary Atherosclerosis by Moderate Conditioning Exercise in Monkeys on an Atherogenic Diet." *The New England Journal of Medicine* 305 (December 1981): 1483–89.

Krotkiewski, Marcin. "Effects of Long-Term Physical Training on Body Fat, Metabolism, and Blood Pressure in Obesity." *Metabolism* 28 (1979): 650–58.

Leon, Arthur S., et al. "Relationship of Physical Characteristics and Life Habits to Treadmill Exercise Capacity." *American Journal of Epidemiology* 113 (1981): 653–60.

Leventhal, Howard, et al. "Cardiovascular Risk Modification by Community-Based Programs for Life-Style Change: Comments on the Stanford Study." *Journal of Consulting and Clinical Psychology* 48 (1980): 150–58.

Lyon, J. L., et al. "Cancer Incidence in Mormons and Non-Mormons in Utah During 1967-1975." *Journal of Clinical Investigation* 65 (November 1980): 1055–61.

Mann, George V., et al. "Exercise to Prevent Coronary Heart Disease—An Experimental Study of the Effects of Training on Risk Factors for Coronary Disease in Men." *American Journal of Medicine* 46 (January 1969): 12–27.

Markiewics, Konstanty, et al. "Exercise Effect on Certain Biochemical Factors in the Plasma in Untrained Subjects and in Systematically Trained Cyclists." *Acta Physiologica Polonica* 31 (1980): 325–31.

Menotti, A., et al. "Habitual Physical Activity and Myocardial Infarction." *Cardiologia* 54 (1969): 119–28.

Morris, J. N., et al. "Incidence and Prediction of Ischaemic Heart-Disease in London Businessmen." *Lancet* 2 (1966): 553–59.

_____ . "Coronary Heart Disease and Physical Activity of Work: Evidence of a National Survey." *British Medical Journal* 2 (1958): 1485–96.

_____ . "Coronary Heart Disease and Physical Activity of Work." *Lancet* 2 (1953): 1053–57, 1111–20.

_____ . "Vigorous Exercise in Leisure-Time: Protection Against Coronary Heart Disease." *Lancet* (December 6, 1980): 1207–10.

Paffenbarger, R. S., Jr. "Physical Activity as an Index of Heart Attack Risk in College Alumni." *American Journal of Epidemiology* 108 (1978): 161–75.

Paffenbarger, R. S., Jr. et al. "Work Activity of Longshoremen as Related to

Death from Coronary Heart Disease and Stroke." *The New England Journal of Medicine* 282 (1970): 1109–14.

Pearn, John. "How Long Does It Take to Become Fit." *British Medical Journal* 281 (December 6, 1980): 1522–24.

Pena, M., et al. "The Influence of Physical Exercise upon the Body Composition of Obese Children." *ACTA Paediatrica Academiae Seicntiarum Hungaricae* 9 (1980): 13–21.

Phillips, Roland, et al. "Mortality Among California Seventh-Day Adventists for Selected Cancer Sites." *Journal of Clinical Investigation* 65 (November 1980): 1097–1107.

_____ . "Influence of Selection Versus Lifestyle on Risk of Fatal Cancer and Cardiovascular Disease Among Seventh-Day Adventists." *American Journal of Epidemiology* 112 (August 1980): 296–314.

Polednak, Anthony P. "Longevity and Cardiovascular Mortality Among Former College Athletes." *Circulation* 46 (1972): 649–54.

Pritikin, Nathan. "Optimal Dietary Recommendations: A Public Health Responsibility." *Preventive Medicine* 11 (1982): 733–39.

_____ . "High Carbohydrate Diets: Maligned and Misunderstood." *Journal of Applied Nutrition* 28 (1976): 56–68.

Pritikin, Nathan, et al. "Diet and Exercise as a Total Therapeutic Regime for the Rehabilitation of Patients with Severe Peripheral Vascular Disease." *Archives of Physical Medicine Rehabilitation* 56 (1975): 558.

Richard, Denis et al. "Role of Exercise-Training in the Prevention of Hyperinsulinemia Caused by High Energy Diet." *Journal of Nutrition* 112 (1982): 1756–62.

Shapiro, S., et al. "Incidence of Coronary Heart Disease in a Population Insured for Medical Care (HIP): Myocardial Infarction, Angina Pectoris, and Possible Myocardial Infarction." *American Journal of Public Health* 59 (1969): 1–101.

Siscovick, David S. "Physical Activity and Primary Cardiac Arrest." *Journal of American Medical Association* 248 (1982): 3113–21.

Stalonas, Peter M. Jr., et al. "Behavior Modification for Obesity: The Evaluation of Exercise, Contingency Management, and Program Adherence." *Journal of Consulting and Clinical Psychology* 46 (1978): 463–69.

Stamler, Jeremiah, M.D. "Lifestyles, Major Risk Factors, Proof and Public Policy." *Circulation* 58 (July 1978): 3–19.

Strokes, Bruce. "Taking Care of Ourselves." *Environment* 23 (May 1981): 42–44.

Taylor, H. L., et al. "A Questionnaire for the Assessment of Leisure Time Physical Activities." *Journal of Chronic Diseases* 31 (1978): 741–55.

_____ . "Death Rates Among Physically Active and Sedentary Employees of the Railroad Industry." *American Journal of Public Health* 52 (1962): 1697–1707.

Vodak, Paul A. "H D L Cholesterol and Other Plasma Lipid and Lipoprotein Concentrations in Middle-Aged Male and Female Tennis Players." *Metabolism* 29 (August 1980): 745–52.

Warren, Michelle P. "The Effects of Exercise on Pubertal Progression and Reproductive Function in Girls." *Journal of Clinical Endocrinology and Metabolism* 51 (1980): 1150.

West, D. W., et al. "Cancer Risk Factors: An Analysis of Utah Mormons and Non-Mormons." *Journal of Clinical Investigation* 65 (November 1980): 1083–95.

Wing, R. R., et al. "Outpatient Treatments of Obesity: A Comparison of Methodology and Results." *International Journal of Obesity* 3 (1979): 262–79.

Winter, W. W. "Effect of Endurance Training on Liver and Response to Prolonged Submaximal Exercise." *American Journal of Physiology* 240 (May 1981): 330–34.